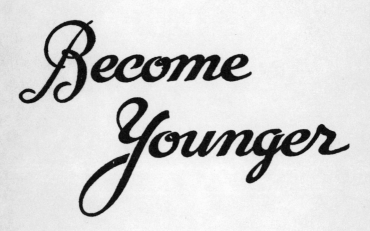

Become Younger

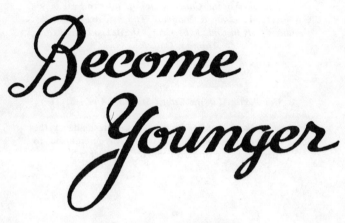

Become Younger

By N. W. WALKER,
Doctor of Science, etc.,

*Member of National Medical Society, International
Society of Naturopathic Physicians, National
Association of Naturopathic Herbalists,
& (British) National Society of Herbalists.*

Published in the United States of America by
O'Sullivan, Woodside & Company, Phoenix, Arizona, and
simultaneously in Canada by George J. McLeod, Limited,
Toronto, Ontario.

ISBN: 0-89019-051-8

Manufactured in the United States of America.

The drawings and sketches in this book were made by the
author solely as educational illustrations. Any resemblance to
persons living or dead is purely coincidental.

●

Copies of this book can be obtained from
your HEALTH FOOD STORE, BOOK
DEALER, or by mailing check or money
order to:

Published by Norwalk Press
2218 East Magnolia
Phoenix, Arizona 85034

Become Younger!

Whether your mind lies close to the earth
   Or whether it soars to the skies,
You will find in this book exactly the worth
   That you place on how high you would rise.

If the effort to climb is too great or severe
   To achieve a goal that's worth while,
You might better stop reading these pages right here,
   And grow old in the old fashioned style.

To YOU who are ready to fight for a change
   From a tired and sluggish existence,
This complete reversal will not seem too strange
   To try out for a while, with persistence.

N. W. Walker.

THE PROVERBS

Wisdom, Righteousness, Fear of God, Knowledge, Morality, Chastity, Diligence, Self-Control, Trust in God, Tithes, Proper use of Riches, Considerateness of the Poor, Control of the Tongue, Kindness to Enemies, Choice of Companions, Training of Children, Industry, Honesty, Idleness, Laziness, Justice, Helpfulness, Cheerfulness, Common Sense.

This Book (in the Old Testament) aims to inculcate Virtues that are insisted upon throughout the Bible. Over, and over, and over, in all the Bible, in multiform ways, and by diverse methods, God has supplied to man a great abundance of Instruction, line upon line, precept upon precept, here a little and there a little, as to How He Wants Men To Live, so that there be no excuse for our missing the mark.

The Teachings of this Book of Proverbs are not expressed in a "Thus Saith The Lord", as in the Law of Moses, where the Same Things are taught as a direct Command of God, but rather are given as coming out of the Experience of a man who tried out and tested just about everything that men can engage in.

Moses had said: These things are the Commandments of God, Solomon here says: The things which God has Commanded are proved by Experience to be Best for men, and the Essence of Human Wisdom is in the keeping of God's Commandments.

God, in the long record of His Revelation of Himself and His Will to Man, it seems, resorted to every possible method, not only by Commandment, and by Precept, but by Example also, to convince men that God's Commandments are worth living by.

Solomon's fame was a sounding board that carried his voice to the ends of the earth, and made him an example to All the World of the Wisdom of God's Ideas.

This Book of Proverbs has been called one of the "Best Guide Books to Success that a young man can follow."

To Promote Wisdom, Instruction, Understanding, Righteousness, Justice, Equity, Prudence, Knowledge, Discretion, Learning, Sound Counsels.   What Splendid Words!

(From pages 269-270, Halley's Bible Handbook, 24th Edition, 1965)

CONTENTS

Chapter 1.

YOU ARE NEVER TOO OLD TO BECOME YOUNGER

Just as you are what you eat, so also you are as young (or as old) as you feel.

Years have nothing whatever to do with a person's age, except in so far as it records the passage of time. One can be old at 30, and one can be young at 70.

The condition of the body is the direct result of the mental and physical care it has had in the past.

I emphasize the MENTAL care, because the state of mind is of vital importance in the condition of every person. One cannot have health and think constantly of ailments and sickness. One cannot be happy and at the same time be wrapped in thoughts of gloom. One cannot be young and be obsessed with the fear of the ravages of old age.

To be young means having all or most of the attributes of youth, health, energy, vitality and perpetual laughter on the lips and in the eyes. It means being genial, cordial, courteous and polite to everybody, irrespective of creed, color or social status. It means being constantly active, with many irons in the fire if necessary, so that there shall never be one moment which will weigh heavily on one's hands.

This is the mental field in which we must work in order to **Become Younger.**

The physical field is more simple, but requires a colossal amount of determination and will power. It means the rebuilding and the regeneration of the body. This is really much more simple than would appear at first, but it takes time, patience and unfailing perseverance.

It is easy enough, after 30, 40 or 50, to say: "I wish that I had kept my youth. . . I wish that I could look at least a few years younger. . . I wish those wrinkles would disappear. . . I wish that my skin wouldn't sag. . . I wish. . ."

Yes, we wish, and wish, and wish, until, in a panic, we rush for artificial means with which to hide "the ravages of age," means by which we deceive ourselves for quite a while, but the world—never.

To **Become Younger,** is that your problem? YOU can do it, but no one else can do it for you.

To **Become Younger** is not a secret. It is just plain common sense and a rigid course of training in self-discipline.

To **Become Younger** we must be **HEALTHY.** This involves far more than merely "feeling well." It means knowing and understanding our anatomy in the same way that an automobile expert knows his automobile.

Do you know WHY you must eat and drink? Do you know the difference between food and NOURISHMENT? Do you know what takes place in your system while you are eating, and for hours afterwards?

Do you know WHY you breathe? Do you know what happens when the air you breathe enters your lungs? Have you any idea of what takes place when you expel the air from your lungs?

Do you know why you need sleep and rest?

Do you know WHY and HOW the body eliminates waste matter? Do you know what happens when waste matter is NOT eliminated?

Have you ever felt tired, weary or fatigued? Do you know what causes it?

8

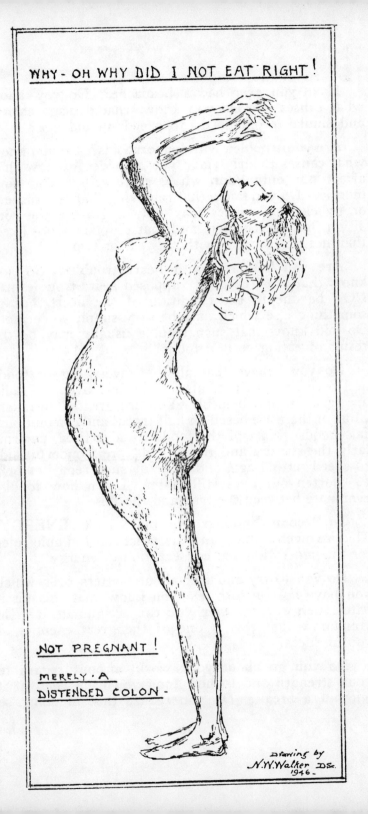

Have you ever had a headache? Do you know what causes it? Do you know what damage aspirin and similar products do to speed up old age?

Are you troubled with hemorrhoids? Do you know what causes them? Have you any idea of how they affect not only your whole system, but also your morale? Do you know that removing them by surgery or by electric needles may only aggravate the condition that caused them and that they are more likely than not, to reappear within a year or two?

Are you bothered with heart trouble? Do you know that most cases of supposed heart trouble may NOT be due to the condition of the heart, but to something else which may be very simple to correct? Do you know that such trouble usually may be the result of eating certain foods?

Do you believe that all the advertising of foods and remedies you read about and hear over the radio are truthful and helpful? You are greatly mistaken. Most of these are based on half truths and conventional falsehoods. Most of the foods so advertised, particularly the starchy and flour foods, are wonderful aids to speed up old age, and most of such remedies help to shorten our lives still faster. Learn how to discriminate between the true and the false.

To **Become Younger** we must have **ENERGY.** This involves a study and the practice of simple rules for the generation and conservation of energy.

Do you worry and fret about matters over which you have no control? Do you know that this dissipates energy faster than you can accumulate it? Do you know that this is one of the great enemies of youthfulness?

Do you go about your work without regard to your strength and to how long you have been at it without a break? Do you realize that in doing so you are literally wasting your energy at the expense of your youthfulness and of your efficiency?

Do you know to what extent the QUALITY of the air in your lungs dampens your energy and induces fatigue?

Do you realize how soon "soft drinks," no less than the "hard" ones, break down the tissues that help to prolong youthfulness?

To **Become Younger** we need **VITALITY.** Vitality is not merely the temporary display of activity, of quick motion or of nervous outpourings. It comes from a deep-rooted sense of rest, poise, awareness and strength which makes one feel "on top of the world" and that life is truly worth living every waking moment.

Do you know what generates vitality? Do you realize that vitality when properly balanced is one of the most powerful magnets which attracts the best in other people to appreciate and cultivate the best in us?

Do you know that vitality can make Leaders of us, whereas the lack of it may soon leave us in the discard? Do you know of any quicker way to become aged, than to be in the discard?

Did you ever consider how vitality can make the plainest of people perfectly beautiful? Did you ever stop to think how quickly such beauty can vanish when vitality begins to drop because of carelessness in the habits of living and eating?

Have you ever noticed how husbands or wives degenerate into premature old people even shortly after marrying, when either one or the other fails to keep up the spruced up appearance that made each attractive to the other when courting? Do you realize what saps their vitality under such conditions?

11

These, and many more questions, have a direct bearing on the problem of how to **Become Younger.** They are all questions to which we must know the TRUE and fundamental answers. Only then will we be able intelligently to map out and to follow a program to eliminate progressively everything that tends to deprive us of youthfulness.

We must learn how to banish all the accepted formulas and indications of premature old age, no matter how old we are.

In order to do this, and to reach our goal, we must study, and there is no better material to study than that which has sprung from experience. To have reached an age when most people have long been dead and buried,—to be alive, awake, alert and full of enthusiasm at three score and ten with the physical body equal to that of a 30 year old youngster is, in my experience, a goal well worth aiming for. Inherently, the cells and tissues in the system of every living man and woman are alike. Therefore, what one person can achieve is well within the range of possibility for every other person to achieve. With this in mind, let us proceed, with an open mind, to the studies necessary to prepare us for the golden dawn of a new and younger life.

Chapter 2.

HOW TO GET OUT OF A RUT

In order to **Become Younger,** many of one's habits must be changed. To do this constructively, one can do it only with an open mind and with the whole-hearted desire to see if it really works.

A closed mind, working against the tide of mental reservations, a mind which has made it a practice to frown on radical changes in thought, habits and actions is the greatest stumbling block towards any progress on the road to **Become Younger.**

Unless one can accept, unreservedly, at least on trial, that which most people would consider unorthodox if not actually extreme, it would be almost better to let life take its course and spend the rest of one's days in the familiar ruts and undertow which lead to senility and decrepitude.

It does not mean that because the vast majority of people have made it a habit of living in a certain way, of eating and drinking so-called "staple" foods and of talking and thinking according to prescribed rules, that these habits, or in fact these people, are right. For incontrovertible proof we need only look around us and see the sad plight of young and old in this day and generation. They follow without question or thought, whatever course is advertised. From infancy, children are rushed hither and yon to have their little bodies poisoned with the corrupt pus and other excreta of diseased animals.

The famous Scientist, Alexis Carrel, states in his book MAN THE UNKNOWN, that injections of specific vaccines or serum for each disease are not very effective means to prevent disease.

13

Not so very long ago public attention was called to the wholesale use of millions of American children as guinea pigs. At 3 months, vaccination against smallpox. At 4 to 5½ months 3 inoculations for whooping cough. At 7 and 8 months 2 diphtheria and tetanus injections. (Let me point out here that Dr. Abraham Zingher, in the New York Journal of Medicine, declared that THE DIPHTHERIA SERUM HAS BEEN CHANGED 14 TIMES BECAUSE EACH NEW SERUM WAS FOUND TO BE DANGEROUS!) At 9 months, 3 inoculations for typhoid. At 10 months the former tubercular test has been subtituted by X-ray tests because of its danger. At 11 months injection of diphtheria germs from diseased animals, known as the SCHICK TEST. (Note: The Schick test originated in Austria. When the Austrian authorities realized how dangerous it was to children, they enacted a law making it a jail offense to use it. Nevertheless, it is still in use in the United States of America!)

These injections, inoculations and vaccinations are usually followed by diseased tonsils, mastoiditis, skin eruptions, appendicitis, heart disease. Sometimes by rheumatic fever, leukemia, paralysis and frequently by encephalitis (inflammation of the brain).

Is this not almost enough to force old age and senility upon the coming generation before it has even reached maturity? How can anyone expect to **Become Younger** on such a send-off, without a colossal amount of patience, hard work and perseverance?

Just look at the manner in which children and adolescents pour poisonous "foods" into their young, growing, undisciplined systems. They grow up into nervous and mental wrecks for whom there is not enough room in hospitals and in asylums for the insane.

Looking at others, we certainly have cause to wonder whether there is not something definitely wrong,

14

in the way so many people exist thru their short span of life. When we look at ourselves, however, we have something definitely tangible to work with. We cannot live other people's lives for them, nor can anyone else live our life for us. This is very definitely our own life, our only real vital possession, and the body in which we live in this life is the only physical manifestation we have in which to function for better or for worse.

There is more truth than fiction in the saying that a man may be down, but he is never out—unless he himself so chooses. There is really no such thing as a hopeless situation. It is the individual who has grown hopeless about it.

There is after all just one formula that we MUST practice if we would reconstruct ourselves, and that is DISCIPLINE. We cannot very well discipline ourselves in the great things of life unless, and until, we have learned that discipline must begin with the small things. Have you any idea what a wonderful feeling it is to realize that thru discipline in small things, the greater tasks that were burdensome actually become a pleasure?

You will understand more thoroly the "discipline formula", as you study the pages of this book. You may even discover that what weighed heavily on your mind as a cross or a nuisance may turn out to be a pleasure or something to your advantage. Any mental burden or cross that we persist in nursing or carrying on our shoulders helps to write plainly on our features the words "I'm heading for old age".

There is a wonderful amount of philosophy in the answer which the little boy gave to the doctor when asked: "What do you want to be when you grow up, sonny?" He replied: "Alive".

15

Little did he know that to be ALIVE means much more than merely to exist. To be alive means conquering every negative condition, rising above worry, fear, sorrow and feelings of inferiority. No one can make you feel inferior without your consent. There is nothing to fear, under any circumstances, once we have learned thru discipline to be self-sufficient and self-reliant. As for sorrow, I am reminded of the Chinese proverb: "You cannot prevent birds of sorrow from flying over your head, but you CAN prevent them from building nests in your hair".

The food we eat and the liquids we drink have just as much to do with the condition of our body as the less physically tangible things we have just referred to.

There is no question whatever about the fact that we are exactly what we eat. There is no other way in which the cells and tissues of our body can be replenished, except from what we eat and drink, and RE-PLENISHMENT is the great law of life.

During every second of our existence, while there is life in the body, cells and tissues are being used up, to be replenished by new cells miraculously created. These new cells can only be built out of the material which we have placed in our system, out of the atoms and molecules of the food we ate, the liquids we drank and the air we breathed.

So extremely important is this question of RE-PLENISHMENT, that its result is plainly visible in the details of the features and the contour of every man, woman and child. It is therefore a very serious problem in our consideration of what we must do to **Become Younger.**

The sallow complexion, lines and furrows in the face and neck, discoloration and lack of luster in the eyes are not attributes of youth. They indicate that the food eaten in the past failed to furnish the necessary QUALITY of nourishment for the replenishment of the cells and tissues involved in this calamity.

Deposits of adipose tissue in those parts of the anatomy where extra fat is neither necessary nor desirable, are also indications that the food eaten in the past was not of the constructive type—advertising to the contrary notwithstanding. Instead of regenerating the cells of the body, they speeded up the degeneration of the tissues and caused the formation of fat. This condition is decidedly unhealthy from the cradle to old age. It is a condition we must try to correct if we would **Become Younger.**

Coupled with the failure to nourish the body with the proper type and kind of food in the past, the retention of waste matter in the system very positively helps the development of ailments and the speedy approach of the appearance of old age.

Waste matter in the body is not composed solely of the end product of the digestion (or indigestion) of food. This in itself can cause a vast amount of trouble and disturbances ranging from headaches to cancer. More troublesome still is the waste material composed of the cells and tissues in the body which have been used up in the activities of the body and which have failed to be expelled from the system.

This retention of waste matter is so very serious in our attempts to **Become Younger,** that we will try to cover it very completely and in great detail a little later in this book. I have found that it is virtually impossible to **Become Younger,** with a body filled with debris which should have been expelled and eliminated years ago.

Thruout this study of how to **Become Younger,** I must impress on you the importance of following it thru with singleness of mind and purpose. By this I mean that every word, every sentence and every fact which is related herein must be studied thoroly without any regard or relation whatsoever to any views or theories which you yourself may have or which others may have set forth. No matter how plausible other presentations of the subject may appear, disregard them completely while you are studying this book. Remember that there are a great many writers and teachers on every subject, including this, many diametrically opposed to the others, yet each claiming to be an authority on the subject. Do not be confused by trying this, that and the other system, until you have proved the TRUTH of the one which will give you the most complete and PERMANENT results.

Only by concentrating on one line of study at a time can your full consciousness and understanding grasp the inner meanings of NATURE'S laws. Anything whatever that does not conform strictly to the principles of NATURE'S laws, necessarily retards our progress.

Therefore I want to repeat that you should study this book thoroly to learn what has helped so many others to regain their health, their energy and their vitality. Having become familiar with what has been successful with others, with people of every age from infancy to 80 and 90 years of age and more, you can then try these principles and judge for yourself, intelligently, why they may also succeed in your case.

Everybody wants to **Become Younger,** but not everybody wants to do more than wishful thinking about it. If YOU want to **Become Younger,** you must DO something about it.

You CAN succeed if you know the Power within you.

Chapter 3.

DON'T ENVY THOSE WHO BECOME YOUNGER
DO IT YOURSELF

Do YOU **really** want to **Become Younger?** Then let us consider seriously the problem that confronts you.

In the first place, do you want to **Become Younger** overnight, just for a short while? It cannot be done, except at the expense of trouble later on. If you want to **Become Younger** permanently, you will have to work at it systematically according to the plan best suited to your age, to your environment and to the physical condition of your body.

To begin with, figure how many birthday anniversaries you have had since the light of day first saw you. Is it 30, 50, 70, 90?

Next, consider the number of years you have lived and figure how long it has taken you to get into the condition that you find yourself in today. You did not get into this condition suddenly, overnight. No, indeed. You are TODAY the sum total product of the food you have eaten all your life, and of the lack of care and attention which you should, intelligently, have given to your body every day of your existence.

You have probably eaten an average of 3 meals a day, as a matter of habit. That means you have averaged about 1,000 meals a year. If you are 40 years old or more, you have consumed more than 40,000 meals in your lifetime, so far. The question for you to ponder over now is this: How many of those meals were actually able to furnish the cells and tissues of your body the real live vital nourishment they needed for replenishment, reproduction and regeneration? Look at yourself in your mirror, and you will most likely find the answer written in every line on your face and neck, in every pore of your skin, and in every contour and outline of your body where it sticks out where it shouldn't.

If the kind of food you have eaten as a general rule is the kind which nearly everybody else eats— mostly expensively advertised foods displayed on the shelves of grocery stores—then consider that you are alive today in spite, and not because, of having eaten that kind of food. Such food sustains life, at the expense of everything in life that is really worth living for. Such food contains no life, and is therefore not capable of generating life, all appearances to the contrary notwithstanding.

We cannot have life and death at one and the same time. Federal laws prohibit the sale of canned and bottled foods in which life has not been destroyed. When you eat any food which has been preserved or processed by heat, you are eating food in which every vestige of life is missing. This may sound strange to you, if you have never stopped to consider the FACTS of the matter. Nevertheless mental and physical ailments, sickness and premature old age, as we have proved over and over again, may be the direct result of eating meals composed mostly or entirely of such devitalized foods.

This problem alone is one which requires much study, if one is really interested in learning how to **Become Younger.** It is truly a most fascinating subject, and when corrected, along NATURAL lines, it can yield benefits and results which the uninformed would consider miraculous.

I happen to have before me the very interesting case history of a young lady. Altho only 31 years old, she awakened one morning in quite a panic. It was a dreary, foggy morning in Southern California, the kind of morning which dispels all ambition from an awakening soul. She had gone to bed early enough the night before, but she awakened stiff, with pains and aches, it seemed to her, in every bone in her body.

In two hours she was due to be at her work and she wondered how on earth she could get her body out of bed. It felt is if it weighed a ton, and every movement was an effort. Her head felt painful and swollen, and every thought that coursed thru her brain was like a dim light which she had to force thru a dense fog. The pain in the back of her neck and across her shoulders seemed worse than ever. It felt like that inflicted by a red hot poker, to use her own words. She was so nervous that only by using all the self control she could muster, did she keep from screaming and pulling out her hair.

So distraught was she this morning that she wondered why she was here, and whether or not life was worth the effort. A glance at her clock, however, left no time for contemplating this subject. She had barely enough time to dress, snatch a hurried breakfast and catch the bus.

She worked in the stenographic department of a large business firm, with a dozen or more other girls. As the bus neared her office panic again seized her and she dreaded the prospect of the day ahead. Her arms seemed to ache more than ever and she wondered how she could operate her typewriter all day. The daily whip of the necessity to earn her living was all that kept her going, day in and day out. At the end of each day she was so exhausted she did not see how she could endure another day.

This particular day in question, however, was the turning point in her life. On arriving home at the end of that day, she was greeted by an old friend, a registered nurse, whom she had not seen for years. This friend had also had her troubles, not the least of which had been a malignant growth which had almost got the better of her. By changing her diet and drinking an abundance of fresh raw vegetable juices, as well as taking many colonic irrigations, properly administered, the growth had completely disappeared.

"But you look so healthy, and even younger than you did when I saw you 6 years ago, I can't believe you ever had a sick day in your life" said our young lady to the nurse. She eagerly plied her friend with questions, in order to discover what could give this nurse, two or three years her senior, so much energy, vitality and radiant health. If her friend could work such a change in herself, surely there must be hope and a chance that she, too, could benefit by changing her habits the way her friend had done.

"It is really a very simple program, the nurse said, but it meant my un-learning nearly all I was taught in my hospital career. The first thing I did was to take colonics and enemas as often as possible. Next thing I did was to eliminate completely all starches and sugars from my diet, and I began to drink one or two pints of fresh raw vegetable juices every day without fail. I drank a whole pint of carrot juice and a pint of a combination of carrot, celery, parsley and spinach juices, one day, and the next I would drink the carrot juice and a pint of a combination of carrot, beet and cucumber juices. I would alternate these juices, one combination one day, the other the next day. Every morning, as soon as I got out of bed, I would drink a glass of hot water with the juice of a lemon in it, with no sweetening. During the day, I would also drink one glass of orange juice—the freshly squeezed juice—and one of grapefruit juice.

"As for my meals, I used the book DIET & SALAD SUGGESTIONS as my guide."

"It seems so simple that it sounds almost ridiculous," our young lady told the nurse, "but I have just about reached the point where I thought I was thru with life. You've given me a lead, anyway, and I want to try it for myself."

Under the direction of her friend, the nurse, this young lady took two colonic irrigations a week and immediately began to feel the fog lift from her brain and mind. She made no radical change in her diet, merely drinking 2 or 3 pints of fresh juices daily and leaving out of her meals everything that contained or was made of starches and sugars. She became acquainted with her neighborhood Health Food Store and bought there a copy of the book DIET & SALAD SUGGESTIONS. By studying this book she was able gradually to streamline her diet, each week eliminating some of the food that was not constructive and adding instead more and more of the fresh vegetables and fruits.

In six weeks, after that memorable day, she was able to eat her meals with relish, having eliminated from her diet all starches, sugars, milk and meat. She also gave up drinking coffee and tea, drinking instead her vegetable juices. She carried two small thermos bottles to the office with her every day, and instead of drinking "soft drinks" she drank fresh juices.

For breakfast, she ate fruits simply prepared, but tasteful. For lunch she had either a raw vegetable salad with some fruit, or just a variety of fruits. Her dinner consisted of lightly steamed vegetables with a large fresh raw vegetable salad with some cottage cheese and some fruit for dessert.

Each day she made it a point of drinking not less than two pints of fresh raw vegetable juices, and whenever possible she drank more.

Up to the day when her friend the nurse appeared on the scene, our young lady looked all of 10 years older than her age. Her work was not up to par in the office, it was considered barely average. She was not sought after by any man, being generally regarded as "insipid".

Within only two or three months after she changed her eating habits, her work was so improved that she was promoted to be private secretary to one of the high officials of the Company. Within a year thereafter she was married to this official. I wish I could show you the two photographs of her that I have here before me, one taken 12 years ago, a year or two before she wrought this great change in her body and mind, and the other taken only a few months ago. The older picture makes her look like a woman of 40, while in the recent one she does not look one day more than 26 or 27.

I have made it a principle all my life that if there is anything that I want to do that any other man can do, I too can do it.

If you want to **Become Younger,** learn how to do it, and DO IT.

You can succeed if you know the Power within you.

Chapter 4.

Do It TODAY—TOMORROW may be too late.

Strange as it may seem, we live in an age wherein we have built up a totally false concept of time. We live 40, 50, 60 years or more to try to learn what life is all about, and when we finally try to put that knowledge into practice, we find that our body is crystallizing. We find ourselves, almost before we realize it, with a body which is literally slipping into uselessness at the very time of life when we could use it to our best advantage.

When we begin to feel the ravages of premature old age creeping upon us, we usually fail to appreciate the length of time it has taken us to earn whatever ailment or infirmity has overtaken us. We then expect some magic miracle to happen overnight by the use of pills or "shots", never considering how long it has taken us to get into that condition. When the first few attempts fail to show the anticipated or "guaranteed" results, we are apt to flock hither and yon blindly following other poor souls in a similar or worse predicament, "trying" whatever remedy happens to have come into fashion.

Impatient to get well or young without working for it, we are usually not willing to take the necessary time to let Nature work for us and do the job successfully and completely.

The result is invariably the same. The unprincipled takes advantage of the gullible until it is too late, or almost too late to make a satisfactory recovery.

How very much better it would be to take matters in hand when we first become conscious that with us everything is not as it should be.

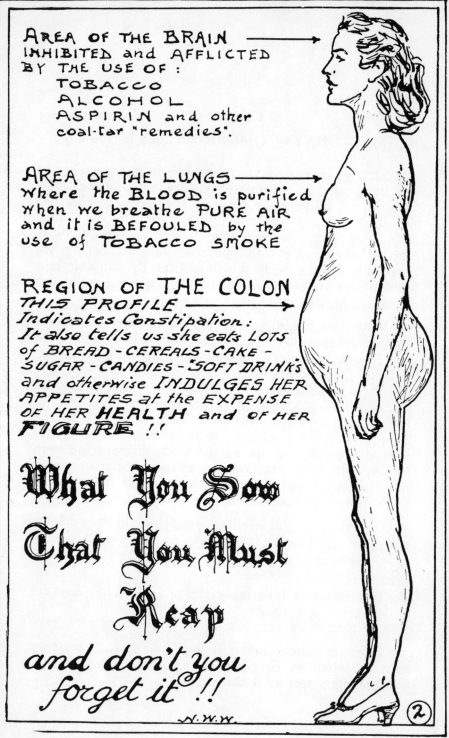

AREA OF THE BRAIN →
INHIBITED and AFFLICTED
BY THE USE OF :
    TOBACCO
    ALCOHOL
    ASPIRIN and other
    coal-tar "remedies".

AREA OF THE LUNGS →
Where the BLOOD is purified
when we breathe PURE AIR
and it is BEFOULED by the
use of TOBACCO SMOKE

REGION OF THE COLON
THIS PROFILE →
Indicates Constipation:
It also tells us she eats LOTS
of BREAD - CEREALS - CAKE -
SUGAR - CANDIES - "SOFT DRINKS"
and otherwise INDULGES HER
APPETITES at the EXPENSE
OF HER HEALTH and OF HER
FIGURE !!

What You Sow
That You Must
Reap
and don't you
forget it !!

N.W.W.

26

My advice to every man, woman and child would be simply:

Read this book today, and LIVE. Tomorrow may be too late.

Study these lessons today. Tomorrow may be too late.

Figure out today just what is the matter with you. Tomorrow may be too late.

Change your wrong eating and other habits today. Tomorrow may be too late.

Begin practicing how to **Become Younger,** today. Tomorrow may be too late.

Base your knowledge on study, experience and considered judgment, not on habit or hear-say. Begin TODAY. Tomorrow may be too late.

Learn to know the TRUTH before you ever jump at conclusions. No human soul is ever in exactly the same state or on the same plane after the TRUTH is learned. He is either better or worse, higher or lower, softer or harder.

There is no short-cut to a healthy, vigorous, intelligent existence. We must do with our body what the builder does when he rebuilds an old house. All waste matter must be removed, and this takes times. The builder can place a stick of dynamite under the house and clear the entire lot in the flash of an explosion, but what would he have? A devastated lot cluttered with debris for the junk man to haul away. It took months to build that house, and it would take plenty of time to rebuild it.

It took a lifetime to build your body to the state in which you have it today. One shot of the wrong kind can relegate it instantly to the sod from whence it came. However, "dust thou art, to dust return, was NOT spoken of the soul." If we want our soul to

27

continue in a pleasant habitation we must take all the time necessary to cleanse our body, first of all. Then, and also at the same time, we must nourish it with such food as will replenish and regenerate the cells and tissues of our body.

We have often and amply demonstrated that age is no criterion when the individual is determined to get well and to **Become Younger.**

For a year we had a Sanitarium under our wing. Our patients were placed on a very rigid program with the admonition: take it or leave it. They ate only fresh raw vegetables and fruits, some cottage cheese, and nuts, properly balanced and attractively prepared, and they drank only the fresh raw vegetable and fruit juices which were prepared in the Juice room of the Sanitarium with a Norwalk Triturator and Hydraulic Press.

One day in the late fall an old gentleman, 87 years of age, came as a guest, accompanied by his nurse. His history indicated that he had suffered with prostate trouble for more than 25 years, while during the preceding 12 months his trouble was so seriously aggravated that he was compelled to have this nurse accompany him wherever he was and wherever he went. On every occasion, day or night, that he needed to empty his bladder, the nurse had to insert a catheter to relieve him.

When the doctor in charge of the Sanitarium told him that he would have to eat only the foods indicated, he protested that he could not live without his cereal. When it was pointed out to him that in our opinion his condition was the direct result of eating cereals and starchy foods, he consented to stay for two months and give the system a trial.

At the end of the first month, thanks to the colonic irrigations he received almost daily and to the strictness of his diet, he was able to discharge the nurse, as his prostate trouble had virtually vanished. By the end of the second month he felt and looked 20 years younger!

I may say that this is not an isolated case in my experience. I have known personally a great many men of all ages with the same trouble, and can truthfully say that I have never known of a single one who failed to benefit from the same program under which the 87 year old gentleman regained his vigor and vitality at such an advanced period of life.

I am very certain that if this same gentleman had taken himself in hand some 20 or 30 years ago, and followed the above program to this day, he would no doubt look and feel no more than 50 or 60 today. As it is, if he continues to follow it, I predict that he will pass the century mark hale and hearty.

And why not? Who is to say what the span of our life is? Did not the Patriarchs of old live far more than three quarters of a millennium?

When we have studied our anatomy, our glands and the various functions of the blood stream and the lymph in our system, as I will try to outline them in this book, we will no longer scoff at the idea of people living way beyond their first century mark. The first hundred years may be the hardest, but the century mark, with a youthful body alive, awake, alert and full of enthusiasm is, to my way of thinking, a goal very well worth aiming for.

Whether or not we aim for such a long range program, the important thing to every one of us is how to prevent and avoid degeneration in any part of our body today. How to side step any indication that old age is attempting to catch up with us. How to know what mistakes we made in the past, so that we may not only learn not to repeat them, but also learn to correct the damage resulting from them

It is not enough to acquire knowledge. A whole library is of no value if all the pages of the books remain uncut and unread. They might just as well remain so, however, if we acquire the knowledge which those books contain and we do not put that knowledge into practical use.

One of man's greatest achievements should be his ability to judge. We cannot, we are not qualified to judge, unless we KNOW, and we cannot know unless we study.

Never attempt to pass judgment on something you know nothing about. Never lay yourself open to criticism by saying: "I don't believe it!" It is the equivalent of saying: "I do not know anything about it, therefore it is false". Always investigate thoroly before you judge something to be right or wrong, true or false. Experience is worth more than all the hearsay in the world.

I urge you to study this book in all seriousness, considering every point on its merits after you have proved its worth, from actual experience. Then you, too, will know that you have found a sound and substantial foundation on which to base your plan to **Become Younger.**

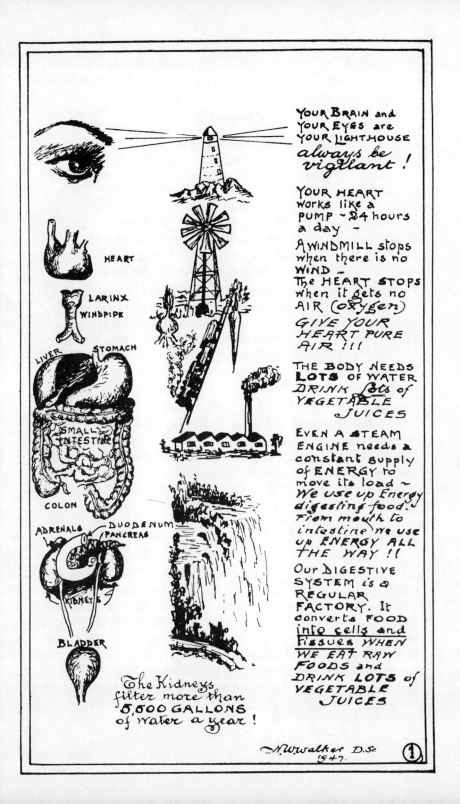

YOUR BRAIN and YOUR EYES are YOUR LIGHTHOUSE *always be vigilant!*

YOUR HEART works like a PUMP ~ 24 hours a day ~ A WINDMILL stops when there is no WIND ~ The HEART STOPS when it gets no AIR (oxygen) *GIVE YOUR HEART PURE AIR !!!*

THE BODY NEEDS **LOTS** OF WATER DRINK *Lots* of YEGETABLE JUICES

EVEN A STEAM ENGINE needs a constant supply of ENERGY to move its load ~ We use up Energy digesting food. From mouth to intestine we use up ENERGY ALL THE WAY !!

Our DIGESTIVE SYSTEM is a REGULAR FACTORY. It converts FOOD into cells and tissues WHEN WE EAT RAW FOODS and DRINK **LOTS** of VEGETABLE JUICES

HEART

LARINX WINDPIPE

LIVER STOMACH

SMALL INTESTINE

COLON

ADRENALS DUODENUM PANCREAS

KIDNEYS

BLADDER

The Kidneys filter more than 5,500 GALLONS of water a year!

N.W.Walker D.Sc 1947.

①

Chapter 5.

IT WORKS!

I am constantly stressing the importance of keeping the body thoroly clean within and without. In my research during nearly half a century, seeking the primary cause of human ailments, and trying to discover means to prevent and to remedy them, my greatest stumbling block in obtaining successful results was the retention of waste matter in the body.

Many times my family and friends urged me, to use their own words, to devote my time to something more constructive than to waste it in this type of research in which hospitals and "Foundations" were pouring millions of dollars. Dire effects on my sanity were predicted, if I persisted in delving into subjects which were anathema to the scientific and medical minds.

When I could see men, women and children all around used as guinea pigs for experiments which to my reasoning and rational mind seemed utterly unnatural, and when I saw these same individuals literally mowed down in a very few years as a direct result of those "accepted scientific treatments" by means of X-rays, vaccinations and inoculations, I was determined more than ever to try to discover the ROOT of our troubles, if it took a lifetime to do it.

From the day I made that decision, I became my own guinea pig No. 1. I decided to live mostly on grain and flour foods, cereals and the like, and I drank quantities of milk. These foods were generally, and also "authoritatively", proclaimed to be the staff of life and complete foods, nourishing foods, foods containing all the essentials for health, strength and what have you. For two years I was apparently thriving on

32

these foods, when suddenly, one morning I could not get out of bed. I had gained weight, rising from 155 lbs. to no less than 197 lbs. There was, to all appearances and by the accepted standards, nothing whatever wrong with me, until that fateful morning when out of a clear sky I was stricken as if by a bolt of lightning. One doctor after another gave me no hope beyond a few weeks, as cirrhosis of the liver, coupled with the excruciating pains of neuritis, were considered definitely fatal.

I refused to take their medicines or advice. I recalled my talk, a few years back, with a friend with whose wisdom I was deeply impressed. He was a strict vegetarian and told me: "If you should get sick, unable to get up, don't under any circumstances take any drugs, they are poison. Don't eat any food for 3 days, as sickness is the result of the retention of waste matter in your body. Just drink a glass of pure water every half hour or so every day, for 3 days and you will get well".

His remarks struck me forcibly while I lay helpless on my back and I thought I had nothing to lose and probably much to gain by doing so. He was right.

In 3 days I was up and around. On the 3rd day, after taking a high enema my elimination was so copious and putrid that I then realized what my friend meant, that sickness is the result of the retention of waste in the body.

I wondered how so much debris could enter and remain in my body. I ate anything and everything that appealed to me, and I became sick. My friend was a vegetarian and healthy as all outdoors. He ate only raw vegetables and fruits, why should I not do the same? I did, and in 6 months I was full of energy and ambition. I began to research on the relative value of fresh raw foods and when they were cooked. When I ate my vegetables raw, I felt well and ambitious and my bowel movements were quite good. Every time I ate these vegetables cooked I slowed down perceptibly the next day, my mind was less alert and my bowel elimination decidedly less efficient.

I again got to wondering. What was there in raw vegetables that caused me to improve so rapidly? I took some carrots and grated them, I squeezed the moisture and discovered how much juice there was in them. For nearly a week I did little more than "play" at grating and squeezing vegetables and realized that I was drinking daily as much as a gallon or more of the fresh raw carrot juice I was "playing" with.

Doctors had told some of my friends that I could not live more than perhaps a few weeks, yet there I was, walking around, as yellow of skin as an Egyptian, yet healthy as could be. Not one of my friends could be induced.even to try drinking my juices! It did not take too long for the skin discoloration to disappear, once my liver and gall bladder were in better shape. I learned that the discoloration resulted from bile and other waste matter dissolved from the liver and gall bladder during the process of cleansing and regeneration resulting from the abundant drinking of carrot juice.

For a month or so, in my enthusiasm I was supplying juices to bed-ridden men and women (at my expense) under the supervision of a Doctor friend who was tolerant, if not sympathetic, of my theories. The results were excellent, particularly when the patients took to the raw vegetable and fruit diet.

Of course at that time I was a very young man who knew all the answers. (Did you ever know one who didn't?) I needed money and became engrossed in trying to make a fortune. This soon became my all encompassing obsession and, as is the way of all flesh, in the course of 2 or 3 years my enthusiastic research and its results not only took a back seat, but in about 4 or 5 years that work might just as well never have been done. Such is the brevity of the memory of an ambitious young man wallowing in the paths of "big business".

The outcome? Just natural, and what you would expect. A nervous breakdown right at the threshold of the achievement of my ambition. The Doctor, in London, England, where my activities were at the time, came to my apartment and told me that my ambitious career was either at an end, if I did not take time and discipline for the next year or so with the hope of recovering, or if I went abroad and abandoning all activities, took a complete rest, in about 9 or 12 months I might be able to get back into business.

Examining my room, the Doctor saw a woodland picture on my desk. He asked what it was. I told him it was a pen and ink enlargement of a 35 millimeter snapshot I had taken in Brussels about a year earlier. Then I had to confess to him that for the best part of the preceding 9 or 10 months I frequently enjoyed myself making that enlargement, often working until 3 o'clock in the morning. Ah, he said, your trouble is not only business and diet, it is also due to lack of rest and sleep over too prolonged a period of time.

Knowing that I spoke French fluently, he suggested I clear up my affairs in London and, instead of starting with a long ship cruise, as he originally had suggested, that I go down to Brittany in the North of France and board with some peasant farmer and eat the food they grew, as they prepared it.

This is what I did. I stored my belongings and packed my things for a prolonged stay in France. I spent a couple of days looking around Dinan and St. Brieuc but these were too large for my purpose. A cab driver drove me around and when we got to the village of Pontivy, on its outskirts, I found a charming old couple with a "family farm" who would be glad to accommodate me for about $2.00 a week (in French money, of course.) They were within comfortable walking distance of the village of some 400 or 500 inhabitants — I expect it has grown to be quite a City by now — and not too far from the Aulne River where I could do some fishing.

This delightful old couple ate mostly raw vegetables

and fruits from their garden, which suited me fine. On Sundays they killed one of their roosters or some other bird, occasionally fish fresh from the River. I was thoroughly enjoying my "dolce far niente" - sweet doing nothing - life and noticed some improvement in my strength. One morning, while Madame was preparing vegetables and peeling carrots, I noticed how moist they were, when peeled. In my subconscious mind something flashed, and I asked Madame, that afternoon, for permission to pick and grind some carrots. Undoubtedly she thought this was a queer British idea, but she gladly consented. I ground half a dozen and squeezed the juice through one of her nice clean linen dish towels. This method was so easy that, unmindful of my previous experience some years earlier, I obtained my first introduction to a cupful of excellent carrot juice made in a matter of seconds. Each day thereafter I assumed the job of making juices for myself and for them. This really did speed up my body building and my health to such a degree that instead of the nine months or more prescribed by the Doctor, I felt well and strong enough to return to London. Needless to say my Doctor was amazed to see me and to see how well I looked. Needless to say, he was dumbfounded to learn my method of recovery. He considered my 8 weeks' recovery phenomenal.

Since these episodes in my young life, I have advocated a raw vegetable and fruit diet with an abundance of fresh raw vegetable juices, whenever possible. I have seen people in every conceivable state of health and sickness benefit from the dual program of internal bathing by means of high enemas and colonic irrigations and this properly prepared and balanced raw food diet.

I can truthfully say that without exception every one I have ever known during the past 35 or 40 years and more who has followed thru with such a program has not only been able to help overcome his or her ailments, but has been able to help prevent worse calamities, even when surgery was recommended, and has had the satisfaction of actually having **Become Younger.**

The natural reaction which many people may have on reading this for the first time, is to ask: If this is true and so valuable, why does not the rest of the world know it and practice it?

The answer is very simple indeed. The reason it is not generally accepted is due to the impatience of most sick and ailing people to get immediate or quick results. This program is harder and takes much longer than the swallowing of a pill or a shot in the arm. People have been miseducated to the use of these quick remedies, and looking for quick, tangible results they completely overlook the fact that subsequent trouble in the form of later sickness or ailments may be the direct result of such remedies.

Nature takes her time to heal and cure, but the results are lasting. There never is any manifestation of pain or ailment in any one single part of the body, in which the entire system is not involved. People do not usually understand that when Nature heals or cures, the body frequently suffers reactions which must be borne with patience and fortitude until Nature finally relinquishes to them a healthier and younger body.

When people appreciate this, and understand it, and try it, they learn that Nature wants man to live a life of simplicity. It is man who makes life complicated.

If we would only learn to streamline our life along simple lines, it would be much easier for us to learn how to **Become Younger.**

Chapter 6.

STARCHES AND GRAINS.

It is not my intention to frighten my readers and students into the feeling that unless they change their eating habits suddenly, they are doomed to perdition. Nor is anything further from my mind than that.

In the first place, most people have not suffered enough to be ready to make so drastic a change, overnight. Nor is it necessary to do so.

If we would **Become Younger,** however, it is certainly, in my opinion and experience, most essential that we do something about the cleansing of the interior of our midriff. In order to understand this angle of our program it is best to make a brief survey of the processes which the foods we eat have to go thru, either to be digested and so become nourishment for the cells and tissues in our body, or poisons we must fight.

It is a painful oversight, on the part of our educators, to have omitted the complete study of the human anatomy from our elementary teachings. I have maintained for years, that children should be taught EVERYTHING about their bodies, inside and out, even before they are taught their 3 R's. They would then learn how extremely important, thruout life, is the care of the body. They would learn that when the body is properly nourished as Nature intended it to be, they would develop into much more intelligent and useful citizens, because their faculties would be more alert and clear. They would learn that it will be their own fault if they become aged, useless and decrepit prematurely. They would also learn that there is nothing mysterious in the cause of sickness and disease, and that Nature has furnished us with all the means to prevent these thruout our life.

They would learn to grow with an appreciation of all life. They would grow to loathe and abhor the very thought of injury to animals as well as to human beings. They would grow to fight with a vengeance the practice of crucifying animals with disease germs for the production of serums and vaccines, the most outstanding crime of the present century. They would learn that this is a merchandising scheme for the sale of serums and vaccines that does nothing to prevent disease and cure sickness.

Don't accept these claims as the truth until you have investigated them as I have done, thoroly, unbiased and with an open mind. I will try to explain later how fantastic these claims have become.

Had we been trained from childhood, to understand the functions of our body, we would know that our body is composed of millions of microscopic cells. These compose all the tissues, the liquids and the bones in our system. As a matter of fact, microscopic as they are, they are nevertheless endowed with life and intelligence. They respond to the stimulus of the mind, whether or not we are conscious of this. They are our servants in every conceivable respect. Like servants in our every day life, they must have nourishment in order to carry on their work. Even servants in our homes, offices and factories cannot work if they are starving, and on the other hand the quality of their work is generally in direct relation to the quantity and quality of the food they are allowed to have.

In the case of our bodies, Nature has endowed our bodies with a vast amount of latitude and tolerance in regard to the care that we give to these little servants, our cells. When the limit of such tolerance, whether in the matter of work or of nourishment, has been reached, we are warned in an indirect manner. We may become tired and fatigued. We may develop headaches, pains or any one or more of the ailments listed in the medical encyclopedias. If thru ignorance or neglect we disregard these warnings, Nature simply slaps us down with a definite sickness or disease.

Such conditions arise directly from the state and environment of the cells in our body. If we have failed to eat food that would nourish these cells, and at the same time failed to cleanse the body of accumulated waste, we have not only starved them, but we have also afflicted them with poisons which the body absorbs from the accumulated debris in the system.

It has been my experience, like that of a great many others, that these little cells must have live, vital nourishment. The food furnishing such nourishment, furthermore, must be of such a nature that the digestive processes can separate and segregate the atoms and molecules composing it so that the blood stream and the lymph can carry them to these cells.

Therefore, irrespective of whatever else we choose to eat and drink, if we are at all intelligent and understand this principle of cell nourishment, we will make it a regular habit to eat every day at least a sufficient amount of live food for the care of the cells and tissues in our system. I will explain a little later why the fresh raw vegetable juices are the finest, best and quickest means of nourishment for this purpose. If we can drink one or two pints of such juices every day, we will derive a colossal amount of benefit from them, if not immediately, certainly in course of time. If such juices are not available, then at least some fresh raw vegetables will help.

I may say here that the vegetable juices are the builders of the body, while the fruit juices are the cleansers. We must therefore bear in mind that the fruit juices do not take the place of the vegetable juices, nor do they have the same constructive effect on the system. Furthermore I want to emphasize the fact that all these juices must be RAW in order to be vital and of constructive value. When juices have been canned, processed, preserved or pasteurized, their life principle has been extinguished and their vital value destroyed.

Atoms and molecules are the smallest particles into which matter can be broken down for practical purposes. Vegetables and fruits are composed of atoms and molecules. When two or more atoms are joined together they become a molecule. Thus the chemical formula of water is H_2O, meaning that the smallest particle of water is composed of 2 atoms of hydrogen and one atom of oxygen. The formula of the starch molecule is $C^6H^{10}O^6$, meaning that it is composed of 6 atoms of carbon, 10 atoms of hydrogen and 6 atoms of oxygen.

The interesting thing about the starch molecule is that it is not soluble in water, alcohol or ether. When I first realized this fact I immediately discovered why the grain and starchy foods I had eaten in such quantities caused such impactions in the liver as to cause it to harden like a piece of board. It also gave me the clue as to why gravel and stones formed in the gall bladder and the kidneys, why the blood coagulated unnaturally in the blood vessels and capillaries and formed hemorrhoids, tumors, cancers and other disturbances thruout the system.

A careful study of the subject also revealed to me why so many people who are habitual consumers of white bread, cereals and other flour and starchy foods have pimples and other and more serious skin blemishes.

I found that, as the starch molecule is not soluble in water, it travels thru the blood and lymph streams as a solid molecule which the cells, tissues and glands of the body cannot utilize. Therefore the body tries to expel it. As the eliminative organs become afflicted with an accumulation of these molecules as a lining of their walls, like plaster on the walls of a room, they cannot be expelled thru these channels. The next best means of exit is thru the pores of the skin and so we have pimples. Here again Nature has provided us with help. Germs propagate more freely on starchy matter than on almost any other. Consequently they help us by breaking down an accumulation of starch molecules into pus substances which are more easily expelled thru the skin, and so we have the genesis of the pimple.

With this picture in mind, you can perhaps more readily appreciate my claim that no system of healing can be permanently effective until the eliminative organs have been thoroly cleansed of accumulated waste matter and at the same time all grain and starchy foods have been eliminated from one's diet.

To the orthodox minded, this may no doubt sound extremely drastic and radical in the face of the fact that for thousands of years people have been existing on grain and starchy foods. My answer to such reasoning is the conclusive evidence that when ailing people, from birth to senility, have been trained to eat no more grain or starchy foods, to cleanse the end product of their eating habits of the past which was allowed to accumulate in the system, and to eat and drink only foods which are live and vital, they not only improve their physical and mental conditions, but usually completely banish most if not all of their erstwhile ailments.

Furthermore, have you noticed how, in the course of time, the skin of people who have been heavy consumers of starchy and grain foods, shrinks, dries up and withers?

The claims that starchy and grain foods furnish all that a boy needs to become a champion and a girl a moving picture star, are based on half truths and conventional falsehoods. If you need any proof of this fact, just look around the lunch counters of drug stores, soft drink and ice cream parlors and count the number of children and adolescents whose faces are a mess with pimples, boils, eczema and other skin eruptions and blemishes. I am sure that you will find invariably that they eat starches almost in preference to any other food. Such is the effect of mis-education.

If these youngsters could only look ahead a few years, they would learn to curb their appetites and eat and drink only those foods which in later years would enable them to **Become Younger,** and to be more attractive, dynamic and successful.

Chapter 7.
SUGAR, CANDY, ETC.

You may have been shocked by the revelation of the effect of grain and starchy foods on the human system. This chapter on the effect of sugar and candy will not be such a jolt. Most people are beginning to be educated to the fact that sugar, candy and similar sweets are really harmful. Diabetes has made such a devastating inroad into the health of children, no less than of adults, that the warning to cut down the use of these items has been generally broadcast.

Nevertheless, the warning seems to go in one ear, and out of the other without registering any sign of danger until diabetes or some other disturbance makes its appearance.

When we eat sugar in any shape or form, in food, in candy or in liquids, it ferments in the system causing the formation of acetic acid, carbonic acid and alcohol.

Acetic acid is a powerful destructive acid, as witness its use to burn warts off the skin. If it burns so destructively on the surface of the skin, I shall leave you to figure out the damage it does to the delicate membranes in the intestinal tract. As a matter of fact its effect is very pronounced as it rapidly penetrates the system. Because of its affinity for the fats in the nerve texture it reacts on the nerves with paralyzing consequences.

The alcohol is equally destructive, and even more devastating, as it acts as a solvent for elements in the body which are only soluble in alcohol and are difficult to rebuild. It tends to destroy more or less gradually the texture of the kidneys. It affects the nerves which are closely related to the brain and has the tendency to disrupt the functions of observation, concentration and locomotion, in exactly the same manner that alcoholic beverages do, but of course more slowly.

When we eat sugar, or drink liquids containing it, as in "soft drinks", for example, the effect on the Pancreas is exceedingly harmful. The Pancreas is the most active of our digestive glands, nestling in the duodenum or second stomach with a duct leading into the center of it. Thru this duct it injects into the duodenum the necessary digestive juices to enable us to digest several kinds of food at one and the same time. When we eat or drink anything with sugar in it, the Pancreas is both overworked and subject to disturbing reactions. This is particularly the case because sugar is a "dead", processed product, and the resulting disturbance is the cause of many ailments and afflictions. It can be accurately said that sugar is a drug in the system, and people who use much of it go thru the same degeneration, sooner or later, that a drug addict goes thru.

When speaking of the destructive effect of sugar, I refer to the manufactured product. In this category we class the white, brown, raw and every other kind including molasses and maple sugar. They have all been processed with heat. The white sugar is the most destructive and degenerating of all, because it is usually "refined" with the use of sulphuric acid.

The only sugars that are of any value to the human system are the natural sugars found in raw fruits, and of course, honey. All fruits and many vegetables, when raw, contain natural sugars, known as fruit sugar.

The processed sugar is particularly harmful to the teeth. Children who are allowed to eat candy in any form have much to blame their elders for, when their teeth begin giving them trouble in later years. Pyorrhea, for example, does not come upon us all of a sudden. It is the product of insidious, slow degeneration of the gums and teeth due to the excessive use of sugar and starchy foods over the preceding years.

In one of my classes in Los Angeles, for example, a lady spoke up who was troubled with an abscessed tooth. She was one of my regular students, and during the lesson on the care of the teeth she stood up and told us she had an appointment with the dentist the next day to have a tooth extracted because of a painful abscess. She asked what I would do in her place. I told her I would cancel my appointment with the dentist and make one for a colonic irrigation with someone who could give me a good one, instead. When I saw her two years later, she told me that is exactly what she did. Her pain vanished shortly after the colonic and the abscess disappeared completely. That of course was perfectly natural, because the abscess was the body's attempt to expel waste matter from the system. Once the lower intestines were thoroly cleaned out, the pollution found its way out of the system thru that particular channel instead of breaking thru the gums.

Sugar is not only harmful in itself, but when used with fruits of every kind it destroys their value. Fruits are cleansers of the body, and even those which are acid to the taste have an alkaline reaction in the system, provided of course they are ripe. When sugar is added, however, the chemical action of their digestion is entirely changed and they generate excessive acids in the body.

By carefully considering this material I have given you to ponder over, you will appreciate exactly why we completely avoid all manufactured sugars, all foods and liquids containing them, and all candies in our determination to **Become Younger.**

When we have need for sweetening, we use honey which has been extracted from the honeycomb without excessive heat. Honey is a pre-digested sweet or carbohydrate which can be used with any fruit or other food.

When we feel an urge for something sweet, we eat dates, or figs, raisins and other fruits rich in the natural sugars.

When a candy bar, for example, is offered to us, we refuse it firmly, as we know that the health claims made for it are not based on fact and that by eating it we would only be injuring ourselves. Furthermore, if we ate it, eventually it would prove to us that the appeasing of a sweet tooth is certainly not the way to **Become Younger.**

We often hear of trainers giving athletes sugar just before an athletic event. The purpose of this is to give the individual an extra shot of energy. Both the trainer and the athlete, in such cases, do not realize what happens after the "energy" effect of the sugar is dissipated. As a rule, the athlete is completely exhausted and often collapses at the end of the event. The reason for this is that the body was whipped into activity by the false stimulant which acted as an explosive. It was just like putting gasoline in an oil stove because gasoline contains more heat units or calories. The result is a destructive explosion.

I was visiting some friends in the East some years ago, whose home was on the banks of a river where college students practiced for their sculling (rowing) races. I became acquainted with one of the trainers and suggested that at the races he give each man on his team a tablespoonful of honey just before the start.

47

He did so. The race was a close one, but while the other team happened to win by a narrow margin, every member on the opposing team collapsed at the end of the race, while every one of the members of his team was able to row back to the clubhouse! The trainer on the opposing team had given each member of his crew 3 lumps of white sugar.

Let us use thought and intelligence before we swallow anything at all that we put into our mouth or into our system. Eternal vigilance is the one-way ticket on how to **Become Younger.**

Chapter 8.
PROTEINS

When people who do not know my eating habits learn that I do not eat any meat, fish or fowl, they ask: Where do you get your PROTEIN. I think this is one of the questions most frequently raised when the matter of Vegetarians is discussed. It shows how vast the lack of knowledge is concerning the rebuilding of the cells and tissues of the body. It also proves that people have no conception of the effect that the digestion of concentrated proteins, such as meat, has on the health and longevity of the individual.

So important did this subject become, that in the revised and enlarged edition of my book DIET & SALAD SUGGESTIONS issued in 1947, I went quite fully into the matter of PROTEIN and AMINO ACIDS. To avoid repeating the 12 or 13 pages of that book, in which this subject is covered, I will appreciate your getting a copy of it and studying it. What I say here will merely supplement that material and will save both you and me the time and space necessary for its repetition.

In the first place, the human body cannot utilize a complete protein, such as the meat of animals, fish or birds, as a complete product, but must break it down and disintegrate it into the atoms and molecules composing it. It then recombines such atoms as are necessary to build up the particular amino acids required at the moment, which may be entirely different from those in the meat we eat.

During this process of breaking down and disintegration the digestive system is really working overtime, which results in the generation of excessive quantities of uric acid. This uric acid gets into the body as a matter of course and is absorbed to a great extent by the muscles. Sooner or later the saturation point is reached in some of the muscles and the acid crystallizes, forming tiny uric acid crystals in the shape of microscopic hard, sharp splinters. It is then that the real trouble begins, because the movement of these muscles causes these tiny sharp points to pierce the sheathing of the nerves and the resulting torture is labelled rheumatism, neuritis or sciatica, etc.

I had a very interesting experience in this respect as a result of an argument on the subject with a doctor friend and fellow student. One of his patients had developed anemia and he had prescribed liver extract and a diet heavy with meat. As soon as he told me this, I forgot all my diplomacy and blurted out: "Ye Gods, man, she'll develop Bright's disease from the liver extract and neuritis or rheumatism from the meat." Needless to say he ridiculed the very thought of it, as the patient's blood count was improving to his entire satisfaction. I asked him to keep a careful record of the case for at least 5 years, which he promised to do.

In less than 3 years rheumatic pains made their appearance and the following year indications of Bright's disease, the breaking down of the kidneys, became manifest. Such proof of course was incontrovertible, as she was his patient and I had never seen her. However, he consented to "experiment" with cleansings by enemas and colonics. He prescribed the diet which we worked out together to suit her environment and mode of living. He asked her to take the juice of a whole lemon in a glass of hot water immediately upon arising first thing in the morning, again in the middle of the day and in the middle of the afternoon, between meals. He urged her to drink as much fresh raw vegetable juices every day as she could consume. She drank one or two pints of the combination of carrot-beet-and-cucumber, a pint of carrot-and-spinach, and when possible a pint of carrot-celery-parsley-and-spinach juices in the proportions given in the formulas in the book RAW VEGETABLE JUICES, What's Missing In Your Body?

In the course of a few weeks he contacted me to let me know that his patient was improving in a manner which was miraculous and astounding to him.

Old age is almost synonymous with weakness. As a matter of fact we often hear people who do not have the strength to do something that is expected of them, asked whether they are getting old. If you do not know it to be a fact, you may be surprised to learn that starches and meat are the most weakening of our foods. The concept that meat is necessary for someone who does heavy or hard work has been utterly and completely exploded.

Have you ever noticed how tired out people feel after eating a meal such as a Thanksgiving or Christmas dinner? Instead of feeling strong, energetic and active they usually want to sleep, and most of them do. If meats and starches were energy giving foods such would not be the case.

On the other hand those of us who eat only raw vegetables and fruits, and drink plenty of fresh vegetable juices, get up from our dinner table always feeling better than we did before eating. Guests who join us at such meals are utterly amazed at their complete satisfaction, and are amazed at finding themselves refreshed and energetic for hours after.

The reason is very simple and logical. "Party" dinners consisting of meats and starches do not NOURISH the body. The food is not vital, live food. The life principle in the food has been destroyed by cooking and the food merely serves as a filler, usually forming excessive volumes of uncomfortable gas.

Our raw food meals, on the other hand, are entirely vital and they furnish the body with nourishment which gives us lasting strength and energy.

It is sometimes remarked that Vegetarians as a rule are not particularly good examples of HEALTH and VITALITY. The reason is that these people have merely eliminated meat, fish and fowl from their diet, but they consume instead vast quantities of grain and starchy foods. Often they cook all or most of their vegetables, and do not drink enough, if any, fresh vegetable juices. On such a diet it is virtually impossible to have a healthy body constantly overflowing with energy and vitality, because the little starch molecules undermine their good intentions.

Under the circumstances it is not right to judge Vegetarians as a class, unless the classification is defined. Strict, raw food Vegetarians who drink plenty of fresh vegetable juices are almost without exception outstanding individuals who are **Becoming Younger** every day.

It is an interesting observation that even when those who eat meat take enemas or colonic irrigations, there is a definite odor of putrefaction on their breath, be it ever so slight. This is inevitable, because nearly all meat is tainted with the outpouring of excessive adrenalin from the animal's adrenal glands. The adrenal glands are little cap-like organs located on the top of the kidneys. The adrenalin that they secrete is so extremely powerful that the effect of an atomic bomb fades into insignificance when compared to this powerful substance.

When a drop of adrenalin is secreted by the adrenal glands into the blood stream it is diluted instantly to between 1,000,000,000 and 2,000,000,000ths (1 to 2 billionth parts) of its strength. This would compare to one single drop of ink spilled into 6,000,000 (6 million) **gallons** of water. If this proportion is greater than you can grasp, then figure that it compares to 1 mile between two posts on a highway, as compared to the distance covered by 5,000 trips to the MOON and back again.

You must now understand how powerful a poison adrenalin is when it gets out of control. Whenever we are angry or filled with fear this gland becomes more active than normal and more adrenalin flows into the blood, depending on the degree of fear and anger.

When an animal is led to be slaughtered he is filled with terror, just as any human being would be in its place. Its adrenal glands pour out so much adrenalin that the animal's body becomes tainted with it. Also, within a few minutes after death occurs, every cell and tissue in the animal's body begins to disintegrate.

The eating of flesh is a custom handed down to this generation from thousands of years of a practice that has no foundation for reason or excuse. Man's taste for the flesh of animals has become a custom, and without attempting to reason whether its use is constructive or destructive he likes it, he wants it, he eats it and evenually may suffer the penalty for so doing.

In all my experience I have never found one individual who had lived on fresh raw vegetables and fruits and used an intelligent amount of fresh vegetable and fruit juices, for periods of 5 or 10 years or more, who during that period had ever suffered with any of the ailments caused by the accumulation of uric acid in the body.

On the other hand, every case without exception that I have had contact with, where I have been able to check the person's diet, where the individual suffered from rheumatism, neuritis or sciatica, meat was invariably a regular part of the diet.

I therefore concluded long ago that if I wanted to **Become Younger** and had been in the habit of eating meat, I would not eat any more of it.

Of course I am not urging or advising that anyone's eating or living habits be changed. Each has the right to eat and live as he chooses. All I can do is to point the way. Personally I have had to learn it the hard way, and most of us have to do just that. I am never satisfied with anybody's experiments, experience or advice until and unless I have tried it myself and proved it to my own satisfaction. THEN, I KNOW that I am right. What anyone else thinks does not concern me. So long as I know the TRUTH, the TRUTH sets me free.

Try it for yourself, see how fascinating a game it is and how much you too can benefit and **Become Younger.**

Chapter 9.

MILK, CREAM AND DAIRY PRODUCTS

The dairy industry has grown like an octopus in the course of the past few decades until today its tentacles reach way into the air, in print and door to door canvass to increase the sale of its products without regard or apparent knowledge of the damage which they do.

Propaganda and miseducation has caused the majority of people to use pasteurized cow's milk as food in the belief that it is a complete food for humans of all ages from the cradle to the grave.

Without bringing forth any preconceived ideas or notions on the subject, let us consider milk, what it is and what it does.

In the first place, milk is intended by Nature to grow the bone structure of the particular animal from which it comes. Thus the chemical constituents of mother's milk are intended to nourish the child for a certain length of time so that its bone structure will develop eventually to what will be needed for a mature individual whose weight will be, say, 125 to 175 lbs. Cow's milk, on the other hand, contains 300% more casein than does mother's milk, and is intended to grow the calf to a maturity of about three quarters of a ton.

The analogy is obvious. The great excess of casein in cow's milk is digested and assimilated constructively by the calf. No farmer in his senses gives milk to his cows as food.

The vast percentage of casein in cow's milk, however, is not digested and assimilated constructively in the human body. Except in rare instances, milk is useless as a human food as it clogs up the system with mucus. This is exactly what cow's milk does. From infancy to old age, the drinking of cow's milk generates unhealthy mucus in the body. This mucus lodges usually in the sinus cavities, in the breathing channels and in many other vital parts of the system. I have found that milk is almost without exception, the most mucus forming food we can put in our body.

Some years ago a little old lady who had **Become Younger** by a change in her habits, who had suffered for years with hay fever and asthma, came to see me in a great state of anxiety.

She had formerly been a heavy consumer of milk because milk was advertised so extensively. When she realized that her ailments sprang from the use of it she immediately stopped drinking it. Instead, she drank daily a variety of fresh vegetable juices and in the course of a few weeks she was breathing naturally and comfortably. For many years prior to her anxious call on me there had been no trace of the erstwhile constant discomfort of those ailments and she was entirely satisfied that she had found the cause of her troubles and had removed it.

Her anxiety on the day in question was the problem of her little 2 year old grandchild. Since birth he had not slept thru a single night and there was not a day when his little nose was not running like a hydrant. Could I suggest anything that would do for the child what had been done for her? The child's mother was all out for the orthodox customary methods of care and feeding. Milk at all times, formulas at other times, and cereals in between. No wonder the poor child was in such a mess!

The problem was to get her daughter entirely away for a few weeks, leaving the child in the care of the grandmother. This she succeeded in doing, and as soon as the daughter was on her way the grandmother gave the baby an enema. A drink of orange juice about every half hour followed for the rest of the day. That night the child slept from 8 p. m. till 6 the next morning without waking up once. It only took two or three days' feeding of orange juice and carrot juice, with some grated raw apple and similar food to supplement the juices and furnish some bulk, to clear up the mucus from the nose and eyes. By the end of the first week the child was entirely normal and playful, cheerful and happy. During the three weeks that her daughter was away, the child received not a drop of milk nor a speck of any cereal or starchy food, nor any cooked food. On her return the child's mother was so overcome with joy that she not only continued feeding her child as a child was intended by Nature to be fed, but she changed her own eating and thinking habits. From that day she began really to **Become Younger.**

In adults the effect of milk is exactly the same. Some four weeks ago I received a frantic telephone call from the San Francisco area from one of my students whose husband had never been converted to Natural living. Milk, coffee, donuts and other starchy foods were his mainstay.

The inevitable happened some months ago when, without any warning, he was stricken so badly with asthma that he nearly choked to death. Emergency measures had to be applied to keep him alive. Under his wife's ministrations he made enough progress to be able to travel and felt he was getting well. He took a trip East but on his return he nearly passed out again. They decided to come to where I am living so that they could get the benefit of my experience in such cases.

I was away the day they arrived and he had to be carried from the taxi to the apartment we engaged for them. That night they had to call three different doctors for emergency treatment, and it was doubtful, in the mind of each of these, whether he would survive the night. However, his wife now had a Juicer and was able literally to pour juices into him all night. On my return the next day he was taken to the doctor who takes care of my friends and students for me when they come here, and was given a good colonic irrigation. All day and the next and the next, his wife continued to pour juices into him and he took more colonic irrigations. Before the end of the week he was able to go to the doctor by himself and the following week he was able to walk the three quarters of a mile each way to and from the doctor's office. Today, only a month after he was practically dead, he is completely out of danger, has gained in weight, walks all over the place and is a decided problem to his wife who tries her best to keep him from over-exerting himself.

This is not by any means an isolated case. I have friends and students all over the country who, by changing their eating and living habits, can testify today to their complete recovery by Natural means alone, after omitting milk and starches from their diet and keeping their "innards" clean and healthy.

Cream is a **fat,** and its digestion is entirely different from that of milk. It should be used raw, not pasteurized, and in reasonable amounts it is not particularly harmful, altho of course it is somewhat mucus forming.

Buttermilk has not any particular virtue in the matter of nourishment, but it is helpful in cases where there is a feverish condition of the intestine. When taken cold one can feel its cooling effect nearly all the way down the intestinal tract.

"Cultured" buttermilk, by whatever name it is known, has proved to be a very profitable commercial product. I have found none that I can consider of any particular benefit to the human body.

I was amused to see and hear a demonstration of a cultured buttermilk at a health lecture some time ago. The lady demonstrating it was not the least bit bashful in boasting about the benefits she was deriving from drinking and eating it three times a day. Nevertheless I do not suppose it ever occurred to her that during the years she said she had been using it, flabby, excessive adipose tissues had accumulated at an almost alarming extent. Her contour had the beautiful conformation of a flour sack tied in the middle, and her dripping nose required the constant flourish of a large handkerchief. This is what we mean when we say that dairy products are mucus forming.

Of course there is no denying the fact that on rare occasions dairy products have been used for definite purposes with excellent results, in case of emergency. When nothing was done to overcome the eventual accumulation of mucus, however, the benefits were definitely temporary, even if they did extend over a period of a few years.

The fact that in an emergency both milk and buttermilk of the cultured variety can be used to advantage is no reason whatever why everybody should partake of them and fill the system with mucus. Pneumonia and tuberculosis are both ailments resulting from excessive mucus in the body and in my investigations I have never found a victim of either of these who had not at some time or another been a consumer of milk in excessive quantity. On the other hand I have never, in my many years of research, in contact with thousands upon thousands of raw food vegetarians, found a single one among them who suffered with either of these complaints.

You may find the information I have given on the subject of MILK in my book DIET & SALAD SUG-

GESTIONS, both educational and enlightening. I am referring to it only in a brief and sketchy manner here, because we have so many more and other angles to investigate in our search for the surest way to **Become Younger.**

You CAN succeed if you know the Power within you.

Chapter 10.

ON FOOD COMBINATIONS

The greatest friends of old age are fermentation and putrefaction. Both these are natural processes of disintegration. That is why they speed up the aging of people. Some fermentation is the result of constructive destruction, but putrefaction is definite degeneration and has no place in the plan to **Become Younger.**

Germs and bacteria were created by Nature to break down and disintegrate waste matter. They are not in the least bit harmful of themselves. It is the end product, the sewage of their colonization in the presence of excessive putrefaction that causes the trouble.

In the preparation of our meals, every food present represents a chemical combination of elements, atoms and molecules, according to a plan of Nature. When these foods are composed of raw vegetables and fruits the elements composing them are vital, organic, live elements, and can be combined in any desired mixture. Any such mixture is beneficial. The elements combine in a natural manner and the result is beneficial.

When the foods are processed or cooked, however, the elements composing them have become devitalized. This applies to all foods.

The starches, grains and sugars belong to the alkaline category, even tho they create an acid reaction in the body when eaten. In the process of digestion, they require the action of the alkaline digestive juices.

The concentrated proteins, meats, fish, fowl, eggs and dairy products, belong to the acid category and require the acid digestive juices.

When the starches, grains and sugars, generally spoken of as the carbohydrates, are eaten during the same meal in which any protein is included, we have a serious chemical situation to contend with. The digestion of the carbohydrates is interfered with by the presence of the acid material, and at the same time the digestion of the proteins remains incomplete in the presence of the alkaline digestive juices. The result is the fermentation of the carbohydrate and the putrefaction of the protein foods.

These results are very definite and real, and not mere fantasy or theory. They have been proved far too often to leave any room for doubt in the mind of any but those who love their meat and potatoes so inordinately that they become blinded to the facts.

There could be no better proof, to my mind, than the case of a man who recently came to this town to benefit from my researches. He was of British origin and few meals were complete for him unless they included meat and potatoes and frequently Yorkshire pudding. About a year ago he had a stroke which was followed within a comparatively short time by three more. They left him bereft of speech and unable to walk. Orthodox treatments in his home town and State left him progressively worse until he decided to come here, unable to control bladder or bowels.

On arrival here, I took him to the Doctor who cares for my students. As usual, the program was a rigidly strict one, of colonic irrigations, quantities of fresh juices daily, raw vegetables and fruits and positively no starchy, sugar or protein foods.

In three months' time he was able to talk quite coherently and walk around a little without the aid of even a cane. His British appetite made his wife's life miserable. He wanted some meat and potatoes. I told him the chances were that if he did eat such a meal, in about three days he would rue the day he was born. Some friends came to visit them the following week end and he begged to be able to join them in what he called "a real meal". "Alright—I said—go ahead if you want to; it's your body and if you want to suffer the consequences don't ask anybody for sympathy. I shall simply come around next Wednesday and gloat over your misery and lack of sense."

They all went to a restaurant famed (only by publicity) for its dinners and he ate a small piece of meat, some potatoes, a little bread and a small piece of pie. I met him quite by accident on the following Monday and he was jubilant when he saw me. "See, Doc., I told you it would not do me any harm? I feel like a million."

I said: "Fine, I am glad to hear that. I will remind you of it when I see you Wednesday, day after tomorrow."

When I went to their apartment on the appointed day, he was writhing on the bed, crying like a child. We took him to the Doctor who was caring for him, for his colonic irrigation, and for nearly a whole hour the gas that poured out of him and the putrid odor of the waste matter washed out of his colon were an object lesson which his wife should never forget as long as she lives. I reminded them both that I had warned them that, particularly in his condition, breaking over the traces would do him no good and the incompatible combination of the foods he was craving would have exactly the effect we were witnessing.

One thing in this life that I shall never be able to understand is the fact that a chemist, of all people, whose intensive education was closely woven into an understanding of the effect of the combination of chemicals, would not dream of the incompatible mixtures, in his laboratory, that he daily pours into his body.

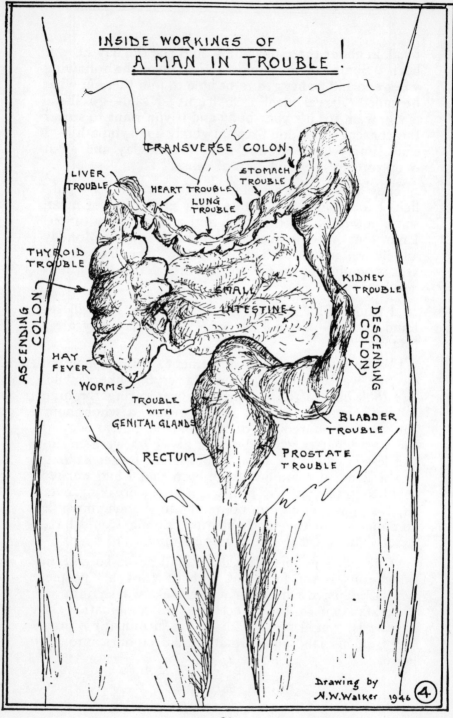

INSIDE WORKINGS OF
A MAN IN TROUBLE!

TRANSVERSE COLON

STOMACH TROUBLE

LIVER TROUBLE

HEART TROUBLE
LUNG TROUBLE

THYROID TROUBLE

ASCENDING COLON

SMALL INTESTINE

KIDNEY TROUBLE

DESCENDING COLON

HAY FEVER

WORMS

TROUBLE WITH GENITAL GLANDS

BLADDER TROUBLE

RECTUM

PROSTATE TROUBLE

Drawing by
N.W. Walker 1946 ④

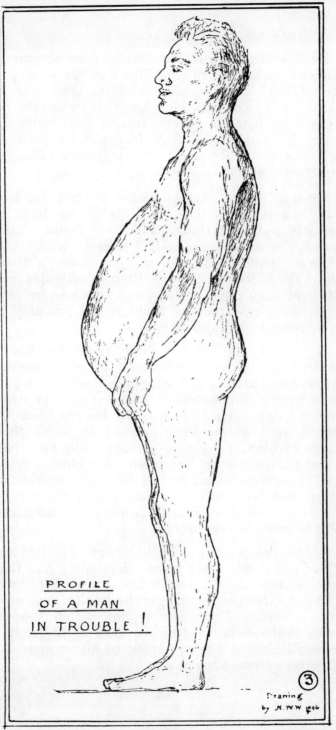

PROFILE
OF A MAN
IN TROUBLE !

③

Drawing
by N. W. W. 1946

I had a chemist associated with me some years ago who had one of the most brilliant minds I have ever encountered, so far as laboratory research was concerned. His profound knowledge of minerals, plant life and chemistry in general was of inestimable value to me. He had degrees from foremost Universities in this country and abroad and his opinion was accepted eagerly in the field of laboratory research.

He was a little past 45 years old, but he looked more than 10 years older. All his life he had eaten anything and everything, solid or liquid that he wanted. For many years he had suffered with stomach and heart trouble, with a liver ailment and a disfunction of the kidneys. He was thoroly orthodox in the matter of health and healing, and I believe he merely tolerated my research, my findings and probably even me, because I paid him well.

He complained often enough about his ailments, but he obstinately refused to listen if I even mentioned that he could attribute them to the food he ate and to the defective elimination of waste from his system. After a 3 days' absence caused by his condition, I almost insisted that he drink some of the juices, that he change his diet at least for a short while and that he go and have a colonic irrigation. He bluntly told me to mind my own business, that there was nothing radically wrong with him that time would not cure, and that so far as his body and his life were concerned it was his business, not mine.

Before the end of the week, however, he had an attack of extremely acute pains. By telling him that in my opinion it might be cancer and that an X-ray would show the extent of the danger, he finally consented to have one made. The accompanying sketch is an exact replica of the X-ray picture we took of his colon, and the profile facing it is an outline of his contour as accurately as I could make it.

66

He disputed every indication that I pointed out to him, and repudiated every conclusion that my experience led me to advance. He did admit, however, that for many years it did not matter how much he ate, he was always hungry. He would not make any change that I suggested, nor drink juices. Less than one year after the X-ray picture was taken, he joined the throng of victims of a system which tries to make life complicated. Even his pallbearers remarked: "I saw him only the other day, and he looked so healthy and strong. Now, suddenly, he is gone."

To confirm my reading of his X-ray picture, I asked that an autopsy be permitted. The lowest sacculation of the ascending colon was a mass of worms. This accounted for his unsatisfying hunger. The ascending colon itself was coated with a thick wall of hard fecal impaction nearly one inch thick, the result of improper elimination of probably 25 or 30 years' standing.

At the hepatic flexure, where the ascending colon turns into the transverse, there were ulcers and much inflammation, which indicated the disturbed condition of his liver.

A little farther, the disrupted condition indicated trouble every time that any fecal matter passed this particular point. This part had a corresponding relation to the heart and clearly indicated where his heart set up a reaction at such a time.

Half way across the transverse colon is the region corresponding to the stomach. Here much deterioration was evident, and we can understand the source of his stomach trouble.

Ulcerations in the middle of the descending colon, the region corresponding to the kidneys, indicated some of the disfunction of these organs. When we examined the kidneys, however, we found much advanced deterioration due to his use of alcoholic beverages, something of which I was not aware while he was alive and working with me.

Imagine, a man in his middle 40's, in the prime of life, with a brilliant mind and the prospects of an enviable career ahead of him, suddenly snuffed out of this life because of his one-track mind and bull headedness. It is a pitiful and a lamentable fact that the vast majority of people simply dig their graves with their teeth, and eat themselves into their graves. This, in spite of the super-abundance of knowledge and proven facts we have, today, that by studying, with an open mind, the simple means and methods which Nature has made available to every one of us, we can, not only defer a premature demise, but actually **Become Younger** by putting these into practice.

I have found that the correct selection and combination of foods is extremely important if we want to **Become Younger.** I have made a valuable FOOD COMBINATION GUIDE which appears in my book DIET & SALAD SUGGESTIONS. Study it and follow it, if you would **Become Younger.**

Chapter 11.

YOUR BLOOD.

Have you any idea how much blood there is in your body? Do you think there are gallons and gallons of it, so that you can easily afford to give it away by the pint? You are entirely mistaken.

The human body contains only about 5 quarts of blood. About 4 quarts of this fill the blood vessels and is in constant circulation.

The blood, or blood stream, is composed of microscopic blood cells. There are between 24 and 25,000,-000,000 (billion) cells in an individual of average health. These cells travel so fast thru our body that it would make you dizzy to figure out their speed. Every 15 to 25 seconds every single one of the cells in circulation, 20 billion of them, travels thru the heart to the lungs to obtain a fresh supply of oxygen and at the same time expel into the lungs the carbonic acid gas from the system. It travels back to the heart, on thru the entire body from head to foot, and back to the heart again. All of these 20 billion cells make from 3,000 to 5,000 round trips thru the entire body every 24 hours.

Every SECOND of the day and night more than 2 billion blood cells travel to the breathing chambers of the lungs to discharge the gaseous waste from the body, in the form of molecules of carbonic acid gas, in exchange for atoms of pure oxygen.

Why do I tell you all this? Because I want to impress on you the importance of keeping the blood stream at its maximum point of efficiency if we would **Become Younger.** From the very speed at which it travels and the vital importance of its work, it is obvious that any interference with its health and activity is going to slow down the system, depress the mentality and open the way for ailments to assail us, **until the claw of old age plows wrinkles of premature senility on our features.**

I would like you to bear in mind, thruout this discussion of the blood, that the entire quantity of blood in your circulation is less than 16 cupfuls. Just visualize that, and think it over.

Every blood cell in the system is a carrier of food and at one and the same time a garbage collector. Every one must have its nourishment to carry on its colossal amount of work 24 hours a day for us, and make 3,000 to 5,000 round trips every 24 hours without stopping, thruout the entire system from the furthest tip of our hair to the tip of our toes.

I was going over these figures with one of my students and I asked him: "How would **you** feel if you missed a couple of meals in one day?" "I guess I'd die of starvation" he replied. Yet, this very man was starving his blood cells every day of his life, and poisoning them while polluting his entire system by the tobacco smoke he breathed in his office all day. He had low blood pressure and was anemic, altho only a few years before he was considered the strongest and healthiest on his basketball team.

His meals had consisted of the regular run of restaurant food. He met a lady in whom he became very much interested, but his courtship brought him no response, until he asked her to give him her honest reason for her refusal to see him more often. Her answer shocked some sense into his conceit and complacency. She said: "In the first place, you smoke, and both your breath and your body odor are offensive to me. In the second place, the food you eat is not helping your physical nor your mental condition. You are already beginning to show signs of aging, which at your age is unforgivable. I am frank to say I like you very much, but I could never imagine myself loving a man who is unclean within, and whose breath would make me want to vomit at the very thought of having to kiss him. It is not only the smoke in your lungs, on your body and in your clothes that emits this odor I can't stand, but the food you eat, the meat and potatoes, the cereals and all that mess makes your breath foul."

He begged her to help him correct everything in him that she objected to. In brief, he stopped smoking and succeeded in having his firm forbid smoking on the premises. He read every Health book he could find until he became so confused by their contradictions that he sought some of the authors for personal interviews. In the course of time he came to me, and found that my program brooked no compromise. He learned that only by treating the body with the utmost consideration and common sense, could the blood cells be kept at their maximum efficiency. Only by eating and drinking natural, live, vital organic food, could the cells be properly and completely nourished. Only by keeping his body clean within and without, could he keep up the complete elimination of waste from his body. Only by rigid self-discipline in all mental and physical activities could he attain his goal: **The lady of his choice, and the knowledge of how to Become Younger.**

The proof that this program not only works but is definitely effective, is the fact that his very fastidious lady friend married my student in little more than two years after the related episode. His wedding gift to her was a NORWALK Triturator and Hydraulic Press, with the wish that it would continue to give them both the health, happiness and youthfulness that he had regained by the use of an abundance of fresh raw vegetable juices.

The object lesson to be learned from this is to disregard the opinions and habits of those who blindly follow what the thoughtless consider fashionable. It is far better to stand on a principle which is clean and pure, than to be polluted by the food and smoke which corrupt, for fear of what others may think. Personally I never hesitate to reject anything that is offered to me, if I know it to be harmful to my system. If the one who urges me to take it, is offended, he or she is not a friend, and I can well dispense with such a one. I find however that to stand up for one's principles increases one's esteem in the eyes of others who matter. Those who deride such principles are thoughtless, to say the least. They live in the tunnel which leads to premature decadence and old age. As for me, I prefer the better, cleaner way which enables one to **Become Younger.**

When principles are involved, always remember that your blood cells are your faithful servants. If you punish them with drugs, "shots" and food which fails to nourish them, and you fail to give them the opportunity to cleanse and to stay clean, YOU are the one who suffers, and it will take you just that much longer to **Become Younger,** if you ever do.

Good, pure blood is like money in the bank. We should not waste it, pollute it nor fritter it away.

Chapter 12.

THE LYMPH.

The lymph is a fluid substance consisting of cells known as lymph-cells, white blood cells or corpuscles, or leucocytes, and scavenger cells known as phagocytes. Every cell and tissue in the body is constantly bathed in this lymph fluid, with the exception of the cartilage, the nails and cuticle, and the hair. Placed end to end in a straight line, all the lymph vessels in the body would cover a distance greatly exceeding 100,000 MILES.

The walls of the intestines are filled with lymph nodes or knots, which continuously and jealously guard the passages into the body against the intrusion of destructive substances and fluids. Millions more are located at strategic points throughout the body.

A specially refined quality of lymph, known as the cerebro-spinal fluid, cushions the brain and the spinal cord against the walls of bone which protect them. The condition of this lymph is of the greatest importance in the mental and physical well being of the individual. It is renewed, exchanged and absorbed, as the need may be, by the tiniest, finest, microscopic capillaries of the blood vessels of the brain.

So extremely important are these two organs, the brain and the spinal cord, that even such simple things as standing up, walking, running, and in fact making any movement whatever, are entirely dependent on their balanced relationship and healthy functioning. The muscles receive their impulses for these activities from the spinal cord, while their coordination emanates from the brain.

73

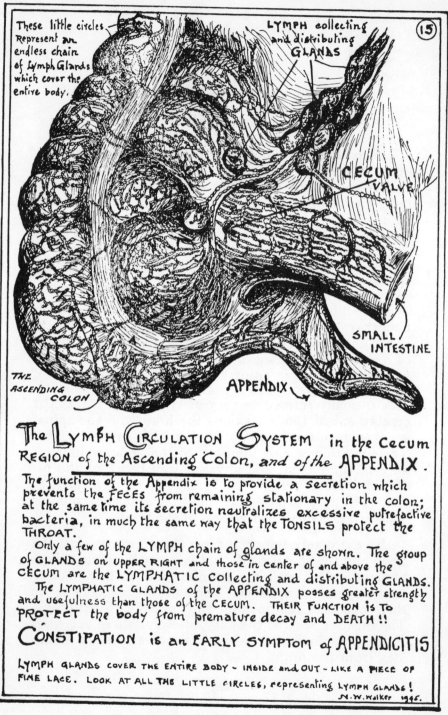

These little circles Represent an endless chain of Lymph Glands which cover the entire body.

LYMPH collecting and distributing GLANDS

(15)

CECUM VALVE

SMALL INTESTINE

THE ASCENDING COLON

APPENDIX

The LYMPH CIRCULATION SYSTEM in the Cecum REGION of the Ascending Colon, and of the APPENDIX.

The function of the Appendix is to provide a secretion which prevents the FECES from remaining stationary in the colon; at the same time its secretion neutralizes excessive putrefactive bacteria, in much the same way that the TONSILS protect the THROAT.

Only a few of the LYMPH chain of glands are shown. The group of GLANDS on UPPER RIGHT and those in center of and above the CECUM are the LYMPHATIC collecting and distributing GLANDS.

The LYMPHATIC GLANDS of the APPENDIX posses greater strength and usefulness than those of the CECUM. THEIR FUNCTION is TO PROTECT the body from premature decay and DEATH !!

CONSTIPATION is an EARLY SYMPTOM of APPENDICITIS

LYMPH GLANDS COVER THE ENTIRE BODY - INSIDE and OUT - LIKE A PIECE OF FINE LACE. LOOK AT ALL THE LITTLE CIRCLES, representing LYMPH GLANDS !

N.W.Walker 1945.

Lymph is the most important element in our maintaining our physical balance. The ear channels are filled with lymph, and their level changes as we move our head one way or another. The changing of this level causes a greater or lesser pressure on the sensitive nerves connected with the walls of the lymph chambers, which in turn send impulses to the brain and spinal column, enabling us to balance the body and so maintain our physical equilibrium.

You can readily see how essential it is to keep the microscopic lymph and blood vessels clean and clear of impactions. Only by doing so can the body retain its resilience, buoyancy and youthfulness. To permit an impaction to form in any of these capillaries would naturally clog them up and interfere with their functions.

What is there that can clog them up? The starch molecule is probably the worst offender. How do we know it? From the fact that omitting all starches from the diet of people who have ailments caused by capillary impactions, and by their detoxicating or cleansing their system as thoroly as possible of all waste matter, such ailments have disappeared after the use of raw foods and plenty of vegetable juices.

If you are not familiar with the results of capillary impactions, I should perhaps mention some, such as blood clots on the brain or anywhere else in the system, tumors, hemorrhoids, varicose veins and hardening of the arteries, frequently dizziness, eye trouble, defective hearing and unsteadiness of limbs when walking, to name but a few.

The speed with which we have frequently seen such conditions benefited when the proper natural steps were taken to correct them, is due to the simplicity on which Nature's laws are based. Cleansing, nourishing and self discipline are the keywords. They are the only means we have found to **Become Younger.**

75

If our appetites are stronger than our will to discipline ourselves, there are of course some compensating advantages. For example, if eating a lot of starchy foods makes us hard of hearing, and eventually deaf, just think, we can still live happily in the knowledge of all the mischief and gossip we are missing! If such deafness causes us to be unsteady on our pins, just look around you at all the tottering old men and women and see all the attention they are getting.

As for me and my friends, we have decided to **Become Younger,** whether or not anybody pays any attention to us.

I must not fail to point out, here, the destructive effect of fried and other cooked fats. Fats are collected from the intestines by the lymph nodes, which however do not collect any protein or carbohydrate material passing thru the intestines. They collect the fats and convert them into an extremely fine emulsion. In this state they pass it thru the lymph channels to the thoracic duct (the main lymph channel in the throat) whence it is transmitted into the blood stream.

When such fats are raw, natural and uncooked as in avocado, olive oil, nuts, etc., and in nearly all vegetables in small quantities, the lymph nodes can emulsify them quickly and effectively, in which case they are promptly available for fuel and lubrication thruout the body.

When the fats have been cooked, however, as in fried foods, buttered popcorn and nuts, donuts, etc., the fat has been converted into an inorganic product and the process of emulsifying it is more complicated. This results in the fat remaining in the circulation of the blood sometimes for hours after eating it, not usable, clogging up the system instead of being available for constructive use.

Have you ever noticed how your friends who are in the habit of eating fried foods, popcorn, donuts and the like, are looking, showing their age much sooner than they should? If they WANT to eat such foods, it will not do much good to tell them what to do to **Become Younger.** But that should not prevent you from following the advice you would like to give to them, now that you know the truth of the matter.

Just **Become Younger yourself.**

You CAN succeed if you use the Power within you.

Chapter 13.

GAS.

Have you ever been bothered or troubled with gas?

The formation of gas is a natural chemical action whereby matter is converted from a solid or a liquid into a gaseous state. When we eat or drink food in wrong combinations, the gas which is generated by the fermentation and putrefaction of such food can cause a terrific amount of pressure in any part of the digestive tract.

I have noticed that children who have been brought up on Natural foods, from babyhood up, rarely have much, if any gas. By Natural foods I mean, the fresh raw foods, not the processed, canned or cooked foods.

Those who are fed canned, pasteurized, cooked and processed foods, however, seem to do a great deal of belching as a result of the gas which forms in the stomach.

As people grow older, they are so apt to overlook the reason for the trouble they have in similar circumstances. The upper part of the stomach is a dome-like structure which is intended to collect such gas as may form during the **natural** fermentation of food. When raw foods are passing thru the stomach, the action of the digestive juices in breaking down the fibers to release the food elements causes the formation of a very small quantity of gas which does not over-tax the capacity of that dome.

When we eat incompatible mixtures of food, such as meat and potatoes, bread and jam, fruit and sugar, a great deal of fermentation takes place and the formation of gas is unbelievable.

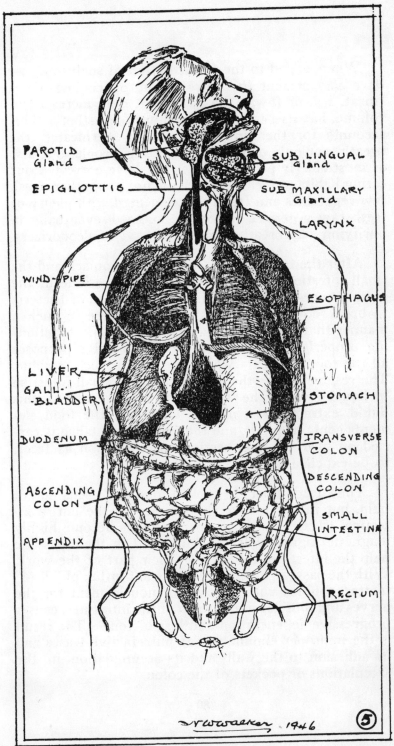

PAROTID
Gland

SUB LINGUAL
Gland

EPIGLOTTIS

SUB MAXILLARY
Gland

LARYNX

WIND-PIPE

ESOPHAGUS

LIVER

GALL-
-BLADDER

STOMACH

DUODENUM

TRANSVERSE
COLON

ASCENDING
COLON

DESCENDING
COLON

SMALL
INTESTINE

APPENDIX

RECTUM

NWWwalker . 1946 ⑤

When, added to the fermentation of such food, we have also present the putrefaction of cooked flesh, (meat, fish or fowl), the gas is not only increased in volume, but its perfume is anything but esthetic. This accounts for the rank odor which permeates the breath, not only of most meat eating people, but also of most elderly people. When we have corrected our eating habits to include mostly, if not altogether, fresh raw vegetables and fruits supplemented with plenty of fresh raw vegetable juices, we succeed eventually in purifying our breath without the aid of deodorizers.

After the food has passed thru the stomach and the small intestines, bacteria work on the residue in the natural course of events. It is the function of bacteria to break down and neutralize this residue in such a manner that, provided the colon is clean and functioning properly, it can absorb for constructive purposes all the food elements which remain in such residue. The residue enters the colon from the small intestine in liquid form. The ascending colon mulches this liquid, extracts most of the water and the food elements contained in it, and the fibrous substance is carried on into the next sections of the colon as feces, to be expelled.

The "dead" fibers in cooked food and meats do not help, but rather hinder the activity of the entire intestinal tract. The fibers in raw foods become highly magnetic, figuratively speaking, and in their passage help the intestines to carry on their part of the work. With the passage of time, the constant influx of "dead" matter, coupled with the lack of nourishment for the nerves and muscles in the walls of the intestines, causes progressive degeneration and loss of tone. The result is the improper elimination of putrefactive waste and its adhesion to the walls and its accumulation in the sacculations or pockets of the colon.

When this takes place, a regular fight ensues and continues between the friendly bacteria who try to neutralize this waste residue, and the putrefactive bacteria who revel and thrive in it. The result is the formation of a much greater quantity of gas than would normally be present in a clean colon.

A certain amount of gas in the intestines is natural and inevitable. Excessive gas, however, can cause a whole sackful of ailments.

I had a friend in New York, for example, who for years had been given digitalis for what his doctor diagnosed as serious heart trouble. He was badly constipated, but would take neither enemas nor colonics, because his doctor told him these would be habit forming.

I happened to be visiting at his home one week-end when he had a particularly bad "heart attack." His family tried to locate their doctor, but without avail. Because of the emergency, we took matters in our own hands and gave him a high enema. After passing the first few masses of rock-like fecal matter, there was an outpouring of gas the like of which I have never seen in any man or animal, but his "heart attack" suddenly ceased. While my friend's amazement was still at its height, I took advantage of the situation to drive him to where I knew he could get a good colonic irrigation. We also had an X-ray picture taken of his colon.

With the evidence before him so thoroly conclusive, he stopped taking his digitalis immediately. Every time he felt a recurrence of a heart attack, realizing now that it was caused by gas pressure against the heart and blood vessels, and not by organic heart trouble, he would take a colonic irrigation if possible, otherwise he would high-tail it for the bath room and take a high enema. In a year or two his "attacks" disappeared.

I have had many salesmen, and others, come into my office, whose breath odor was so offensive I could not bear them within 6 feet of me. It took no guess work to determine the source of this odor. Discoloration around the eyes, a sallow complexion, a protruding midriff and a lack of youthful springiness or elasticity in their stride were sufficient indications to me that intestinal degeneration was working like a tractor cultivating their interiors for the seed of premature old age.

When we permit the system to become progressively and permanently stagnant, we are issuing an urgent call for old age to come and meet us. Old age just loves gas, but few people realize it. Knowing this, we do everything in our power to eat and live correctly so we may **Become Younger.**

All beverages containing alcohol or sugar are gas forming. That is why even a cocktail causes the breath to smell so foul.

When we change over from the orthodox way of eating and living, to the correct natural methods, we must not expect that gas will entirely vanish from our system. Even after we have formed a regular habit of eating and living the way we were intended to, there will be much gas present. This is due to the cleansing processes, in the first place, and this may take years to accomplish completely, but it is worth it in order to **Become Younger.**

Nervous tension is another cause to blame for the presence of gas. Such tension interferes with the digestion of our food and produces gas.

On the other hand it also takes years for the starved organs in our body to be nourished back to 100% efficiency. Even during this period of rebuilding, we will be forming plenty of gas. Its effect however will not be harmful, and certainly not so obnoxious as the gas that emanates from a body which is overloaded with fermenting and putrefying waste to which more is added daily. This merely interferes with the process of **Becoming Younger.**

Furthermore, our very method of living, in this "civilized" existence, without the proper exercise that was intended for man, with air polluted with the carbon monoxide from thousands of automobiles and the fumes from factories, retards our progress. These handicaps are all conducive to the formation of gas in the system, because the body MUST have pure air, sunshine and exercise, besides the right food, to **Become Younger.**

I shall have more to say regarding GAS when I tell you about the cause and effect of constipation, later in this book.

In the meantime, we would do everything possible to reduce the formation of gas in our system, by eating correctly, keeping relaxed and drinking plenty of carrot and spinach juice. We have also found that garlic helps tremendously, particularly if it can be taken in a form which will make it most completely available in the colon itself. We have found that a good quality garlic capsule taken a little while before meals and one shortly before retiring, swallowed with a glass of vegetable juice, has been very helpful in the long run. Only I would advise NOT to **bite** into the capsule! I would swallow it whole. To bite into it might ostracise you socially.

*Garlic capsules can be obtained from your local Health Food Store.

83

Chapter 14.

YOUR LUNGS.

The average bunch of grapes has anywhere from 50 to 200 or 300 grapes on it. If your lungs were a complete hollow and you put one bunch of grapes in it, you would be most uncomfortable because of the space they would need.

Your lungs are like bunches of grapes, only these are microscopic in size. These bunches are so small, in fact, that there are 400 million bunches in your lungs. One bunch could just about slip thru the eye of a small needle.

If you smoke, you have never appreciated the importance of your lungs. Your lungs can keep you young or they can age you so fast that the result would be pitiful. Women who smoke, for example, age years every year that they smoke, and soon it hardens and coarsens them and their features.

Tobacco advertisements are doing more perhaps than any other cause, to prevent people from **Becoming Younger,** particularly those people who are gullible enough to believe them.

To estimate the value of your lungs you must realize that we can live days, and sometimes weeks, with nothing to eat, but only 5 or 6 minutes without air would transform us into a cadaver.

The blood cells or corpuscles MUST have oxygen in order to be able to work for us. They need oxygen to maintain the even temperature of our body. They need it to burn up some of the waste matter in the system. They need it to help break down the struc-

84

ture of the food we eat and the liquids we drink, so that the atoms and molecules may become available to the cells, tissues and glands of the body.

While we only breathe in, about one pint of air at a time, we breathe into our system on an average more than 20,000 pints, or 2,500 gallons of air a day. Every time that we exhale, or expel our breath, it means that millions of molecules have undergone their atom-splitting performance and the resulting debris, in the form of carbonic acid gas, is being eliminated from our body in that breath, provided that there is no interference within the lungs.

If we have been eating foods and drinking liquids which are mucus forming, such as starches and milk, etc., some of the mucus resulting from the digestion of such foods and liquids, finds its way into the lungs. Likewise, when we breathe air which is saturated with tobacco smoke and alcohol fumes, it tends to pack these little bunches in our lungs so tightly that air and oxygen cannot get thru. It is only the fact that kind Nature endowed us with more than 400 million such bunches that so many people are living today. Correction: that so many people are **existing** today. An amazing number of these who are walking around today died when they were 30 or 35 years old, and are waiting to be 50 or 60 before they are buried.

We cannot expect to **Become Younger** unless we make use of all the facilities which Nature has given us with which to get all the oxygen possible into our system, from the air we breathe.

Pollution of any of the air channels of the lungs is the cause of asthma, hayfever, bronchitis, colds, catarrh, fatigue, and many other ailments. This pollution comes not only from the wrong food, but also from the fact that the lungs become filled with debris. The action of our breathing is controlled by the nerve centers at the base of the brain. People who smoke in order "to soothe their nerves" do not know what they are talking about. The sense of relaxation from smoking is purely a delusion and self-deception. It results from the anesthetizing or deadening of the nerves, something that will never help us to **Become Younger.** Furthermore, the poison from the nicotine is bad enough, but the poisoning of the body by the carbon monoxide in cigarettes is even worse. As the body needs oxygen and the lungs cannot furnish it in sufficient quantity because of the smoke and other debris wedged in the lungs, it steals atoms of oxygen from the carbonic acid gas (Carbon dioxide=CO^2) to compensate for the lack of it, as the carbonic acid gas cannot be completely expelled. This leaves carbon monoxide, (CO), a dangerous and deadly poison, as a residue in the system.

Whenever I come out of a room where the air is foul, whether because of the smokers who made it so, or because of lack of sufficient ventilation, I deliberately exhale, or expel, my breath as forcibly and completely as possible several times. If I were to take deep breaths without doing so, I would simply be packing the foul air still tighter and deeper into my lungs, but by forcibly expelling it first, it gives my lungs the chance to take in more pure, fresh air without any interference from the foul or heavier air that had collected in the bottom of the lungs.

As a matter of fact, this system of breathing is very efficient in helping to refresh us, particularly if we walk around, whether in the room, with the windows wide open, or in the out of doors, swinging our arms and legs in rhythm while exhaling and while inhaling. Try it, and see if it does not refresh you surprisingly. It really makes one feel that it is worth while to do anything constructive that will make us **Become Younger.**

Chapter 15.

THE HEART in Youth and Old Age.

"As the barometer foretells the storm,
  "While still the skies are clear, the weather warm,
"So something in us, as old age draws near,
  "Betrays the pressure of the atmosphere."

The poet knew from experience what "that something in us" did to him, and to everybody, when the pulsations of the heart begin to lose their efficiency.

We have, in the heart, a mechanism so miraculous that no inventor has yet ever been able, even remotely, to duplicate. It is about the size of a man's medium size closed fist, yet functions like a pump or an engine 24 hours a day so long as life remains in the body.

The pumping action of the heart causes it to "beat" about 100,000 times a day, during which time it pumps between 10,000 and 11,000 quarts of blood throughout the body. Bearing in mind that the body only contains about 5 quarts of blood, think of the work that the heart does in circulating the blood thru the system in just one year of your life. It pumps more than 45,-000,000 GALLONS of blood in a span of only 50 years.

The rate of the heart beat is regulated by the amount of carbonic acid in the blood. The oxygen which we inhale combines, in the system, with the carbon present in the food we eat and forms carbonic acid. As we have already seen, this carbonic acid, as gas, is expelled thru the lungs as we breathe. It is a heavy gas, so poisonous that if the air we breathe happens to contain about 14 per cent of it, we would die.

In the system it is a waste product, but only valuable when in proper relation to the needs of the body. We have seen that it is the result of the oxygen and carbon atoms combining. Bear this in mind when you think of eating any concentrated carbohydrate foods, such as bread, cereals, and all other starch and flour products. Their carbon content is too high.

As we have seen, the heart beat is regulated by the carbonic acid content of the blood. The more starchy foods we eat, the more carbon atoms we force into the blood, and the greater is its carbonic acid content. As soon as we make a move of any kind, the muscles involved in it produce carbonic acid. Within 10 seconds the carbonic acid molecules have caused the heart to beat more rapidly. The greater the quantity of carbon we add to the system, the greater is the generation of carbonic acid and consequently the more danger of increasing the action of the heart.

If you will study these few paragraphs carefully, you will readily appreciate where all the heart trouble comes from in people who just love to eat starchy foods, cereals and the like. That chubby boy or girl that your neighbor is so proud of is just full of carbonic acid which sooner or later, if the diet is not corrected, may start quite a series of heart ailments. High blood pressure, no less than low blood pressure, is nothing more than the result of eating too many carbon foods. These form carbonic acid which interferes with the smooth and rhythmic function of the blood and of the heart. Sugar of every manufactured variety has the same effect.

With these facts before us, facts which in this enlightened day cannot be contradicted, it is easy to understand why it is so necessary to watch one's diet at all times, no less than the proper elimination of waste from the body, in order to **Become Younger.**

It is truly difficult, when in a rut, to know just where to turn. Yet our wonderful Father who created us has never failed yet to open the way towards enlightenment for those who are ready to take stock of themselves. In order to **Become Younger,** we must have a very positive desire and incentive to do so, no matter how many summers and winters have passed us by.

I believe you will be interested in a letter I have before me, from a man and his wife, both approaching their 80th birthdays.

Dear Doctor Walker:

15 years ago I was obliged to retire, sick in body and weary at heart. My wife was able to do little more than run our household in a haphazard manner. Sleepless nights, fearful hours of darkness tusseling with senility and the fear of the Poor House, painful days of shuffling around with joints and muscles aching with the sting of arthritis and rheumatism, life a nightmare with no light or hope for our remaining days. It was a problem.

Medicines, pills and sedatives had long stopped giving more than fleeting relief, temporary at best, but the accompanying bills for medical attendance continued in increasing volume.

On our way to Church one Sunday, we passed a Health Food Store displaying the following sign in the window, which arrested our gaze. It said:

DON'T BE OLD—do something about it.
DRINK FRESH VEGETABLE JUICES. Clear that waste from your body, that is making you feel old,
THANK GOD that TODAY you have determined to Become Younger!

We read it over and over, then walked silently to Church, each of us wondering whether that message could possibly be meant for us.

Next morning we went timidly into that store and poured our problems into the sympathetic ears of its owner.

He told us that infirmity and sickness, at any age, is the direct result of loading up the body with food which contained no vitality, and at the same time allowing the intestines to remain loaded with waste matter. We were surprised and shocked to learn that our food, which had all our lives been the best, according to accepted standards, was responsibe for the greater part of our ailments and troubles.

Breads and cereals, which were advertised in the papers, magazines and radio as nourishing and good, sponsored by what we thought were reputable channels, and which everybody takes for granted, were what we had been existing on. We were now led to believe that these representations were utterly false and misleading. The store owner was more than 70 years old, vigorous, healthy and energetic, and in the face of such evidence we felt there was no room for doubt or argument. He had changed his diet 15 or 20 years ago, and now ate only raw foods and drank vegetable and fruit juices which his store made fresh every day. Today he looks no more than 50 or 55 years old.

We felt very much blessed, when we left his store with a number of health books, and his admonition not to become confused by the contradictory opinions of the various authors. Just to use that which was nearest to Nature, when it came to food.

I did not mean to take up so much of your valuable time, but I know that you will be interested in the fact that we have been following the program outlined by him for the past year, and both my wife and I feel that it will not be very long before we will be sufficiently "mended" to resume work. It seems to me incredible that the vegetable juices you recommend in your book, are not available as freely as milk, for example. If people could only *be made to try them, as we did, they would realize the new world that lies ahead of them. We ourselves already feel 10 years younger.*

Gratefully and Sincerey Yours,

Every now and again, when one person after another asks me: How long would I have to stay on such a diet; how long would I have to drink these juices? —I feel that my efforts to re-educate people may have been in vain. When I get a letter such as this one, however, a new horizon opens wide in front of me, and I think of the Master's words: In as much as ye have done it unto the least of these, ye have done it unto Me.

You, too, can succeed if you know the Power within you.

Chapter 16.

YOUR NERVES.

Our nerve system is one of our most valuable assets. Just as soon as we relax our self discipline, our nerves respond in kind. They go hay-wire. A young body is young, vital, energetic and healthy just as long as the nerve system coordinates with the functions of the rest of the body. As soon as this coordination slackens, we see old age peeking at us around the corner.

How often have you heard people referred to as "a bundle of nerves"? Their condition may be mental or physical. Lack of nerve coordination as the outcome of emotional upsets would result in a mental state of nerves. Starvation of the nerve system, or interference by debris would be the physical cause. Lack of rest, insufficient sleep, impure air, stimulants, these are all strings that hold the "bundle of nerves" in such a knot that the victim is of less use to himself than to anyone else.

During sleep the nerve system acts as a storage battery to replenish the vital forces and build up the storage of energy. Hence the need of rest.

The healthy condition of our nerves is dependent on the food we eat and the liquid we drink. We cannot afford to have a single nerve in our body "doped" in any way, shape or form, because the entire nerve system thruout the body is dependent on the vitality of every individual nerve, no matter how unimportant it may seem.

A word picture of the value of the nerve system will give you a better understanding of what nerves tell us, as well as what they do.

Every organ, limb and part of the body has three important nerve endings, one is in the iris of the eye, one is in the walls of the colon, and one is in the sole of the feet.

When we take any drugs or anything like bicarbonate of soda, for example, which are inorganic products, and they are not more or less promptly expelled from the body, they form a deposit in some part of the anatomy. It happens that bicarbonate of soda has an affinity for the upper part of the head, the region of the brain. The use of it will sooner or later display a silver-like crescent on the upper part of the iris. This means that the body did not expel it and it lodged in the region of the brain. The nerves in that region automatically register its presence there.

This is but one example of what it would take one or two volumes to cover more fully.

When there is any disturbance in any particular part of the colon, we can tell which is the corresponding part of the anatomy where the affliction is, or is likely to appear. Thus, the nerve at the lowest pouch of the ascending colon corresponds to the Pituitary gland, which is the gland of mental and physical balance. This is where we often find a nest of worms, causing this pouch to prolapse and to become inflamed, which is clearly visible in an X-ray picture. It has repeatedly been proved to indicate mental disturbances and frequently physical unbalance resulting in epileptic fits. This angle is covered more fully, and illustrated, in the chapter on constipation later in this book.

Other nerve endings are in the sole of the feet. I made a chart of the sole of the feet, calling it FOOT RELAXATION CHART, in which I have depicted the various parts of the body which can be helped and relaxed by pressing on the parts indicated. One of my students used this chart to excellent advantage when her father had what he thought was a heart attack. She pressed the sole of his foot at the point indicated on the chart, corresponding to the heart, but there was virtually no response. She then pressed on the points indicated corresponding to the part of the colon below the heart, and gas poured out of his throat and thru his bowels, whereupon the "heart attack" disappeared. Tense nerves had caused a pouch in the colon to tighten, allowing the gas to accumulate until the ballooning of the pouch created excessive pressure against nerves and muscles, resulting in increased heart action. Relaxing the tight nerves helped to dissipate the gas and the heart was able to resume its normal beat.

The main distributing nerve center of the body is located at the base of the brain in a structure known as the Medulla Oblongata, just above the nape of the neck. From here it spreads out to every part of the anatomy. It is divided into two main sections or divisions. One is the abdominal, or sympathetic nervous system, which does not have anything to do with your sympathies, by the way. The other is the central nervous system consisting of the brain and the spinal cord with its many branches.

The sympathetic nervous system gives us the directing force, coming mainly from the brain centers. It affects our breathing, the regulation of the temperature of the body, the water in our system, the organs involved in our eating and drinking, the regulation of the distribution of the blood, the tension of the blood and lymph-vessels, and many other functions and activities.

The central nervous system is the network of nerves which forms the brain and spinal cord. From these it spreads out thru the body to the skin.

When you get a splinter in your finger, an impulse is transmitted by the nerve to one in the spinal cord. This in turn transmits the sensation to another nerve

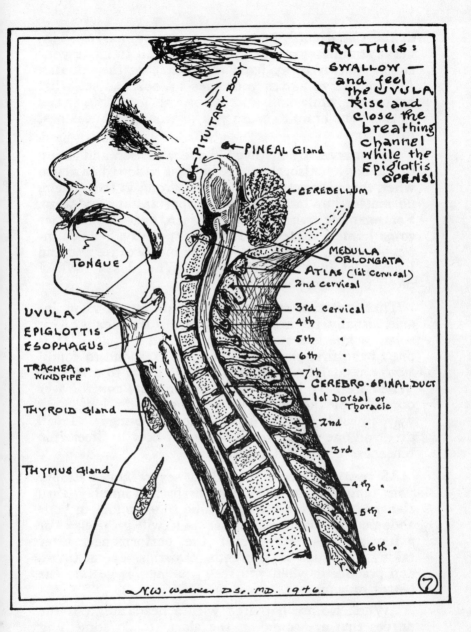

TRY THIS:
SWALLOW —
and feel
the UVULA
Rise and
close the
breathing
channel
while the
Epiglottis
OPENS!

PITUITARY BODY

PINEAL Gland

CEREBELLUM

MEDULLA
OBLONGATA

ATLAS (1st Cervical)

2nd Cervical

3rd Cervical

4th "

5th "

6th "

7th "

CEREBRO-SPINAL DUCT

1st Dorsal or
Thoracic

2nd "

3rd "

4th "

5th "

6th "

TONGUE

UVULA

EPIGLOTTIS

ESOPHAGUS

TRACHEA or
WINDPIPE

THYROID Gland

THYMUS Gland

N.W. Warren DSc, MD. 1946.

⑦

95

in the spinal cord, known as a motor nerve. This nerve stimulates muscles that cause you to move your finger quickly away from the source of the splinter. Another nerve moves your eyes to look and see what happened, while still another nerve gets busy and tickles your brain to cause you to wonder what is best to do next.

The nerves are involved in every motion and action of the body. Also, they are the first to sound an alarm when there is anything whatever wrong in the system, no matter how apparently unimportant it may seem. For example, when we have been overworking, we come home irritated. (This, by the way, I don't intend, personally, to mean you and me, because you and I never let anything irritate us. When I say "We" I mean other people.)

That irritation results in tying us into a knot, inside, usually in the region of the solar plexus. This solar plexus is a mass of nerves and muscles. It is one of the first parts of the body to respond to conditions outside of ourselves which we allow to affect us. When we have learned to have complete control over our solar plexus, we will have progressed a long, long way, towards helping us to **Become Younger.** I will give you one good exercise to learn how to "feel" the tenseness of the solar plexus:

Move your abdomen in and out several times. Empty your lungs by blowing out your breath forcibly, thru clenched teeth, while at the same time pulling **in** your abdomen, or diaphram, as far as it will go. Relax for a few seconds, then repeat the performance, after taking in a good long breath. Do this several times, and practice it when you feel your nerves getting the better of you.

When we are bothered with a headache, it is the nerves that are sounding the alarm to do something constructive to help remedy whatever has gone wrong in our system. To take aspirin for example, merely deadens the nerve to stop the warning. It is exactly like cutting the wires of your front door bell because a neighbor has come to warn you that your house is on fire. Whatever we take to "kill" or deaden pain, numbs or drugs the nerves. It may be alright to give us temporary relief, PROVIDED that we do something to remedy the **cause** and thereafter promptly take steps to get the painkiller out of our system. A headache, may usually be an indication that waste matter in the colon is either clogging up that organ excessively or that it has been allowed to overstay its welcome and as a result is causing poisons to be absorbed from the colon into the system. In my study of thousands of cases of headaches, the colon has been the greatest headache of all, because people will not stop to think, and realize the relation between it and the pain.

A toothache is another warning by the nerves that the system needs a thoro cleaning out—not of the teeth from our mouth, as we will need these as long as we live—but of waste matter that is poisoning the body. Long experience has resulted in my firm conviction that any person who follows the advice to have his teeth extracted because of arthritis, rheumatism, or any other trouble in his body, including abscesses, gets what he deserves, for not using the brain that his Creator placed in his skull. I have yet to find the man or woman truthfully happy with false teeth.

One of the most pitiful human derelicts I have ever known, joined one of my classes in San Francisco. He was a robust, strong and healthy young man when he was drafted into the Navy. According to the rules of the medical department of the Navy, he was given the whole gamut of "shots", vaccinations and inoculations. Like hundreds, if not thousands of such unfortunate victims, the damage resulting directly from these pestilential injections completely incapacitated him and he was shuttled from one hospital to another until he finally landed in one in San Francisco. There they found they could do nothing more for him than had already been done, and everything that had been done made him progressively worse. So the "authorities" who examined him very carefully, finally said: "Well, let's try taking his teeth out and see if that will help." Up to that moment his teeth had been almost the only part of his anatomy which had not begun to disintegrate. Shortly after his teeth were extracted he almost lost his power of speech and was hardly able to walk around. His nerves failed to coordinate half the time and left him exhausted and helpless. You have known cases like this, I am sure, because the army and navy hospitals have so many of them they don't know what to do with them.

Strange as it may seem, one of them came to see me some 10 years ago, sent by one of the Veteran's Hospitals. He was so nervous and exhausted when he came into my office he could hardly walk across the room to sit down. He was suffering from cancer, according to the report, and our analyses led me to the conclusion that it resulted from army vaccination and inoculations. So bad was his case that, even tho they sent him to me, they notified his family in the middle West to send somebody, very soon, to take his body home. He was only about 28 years old, far too young for conversion into a cadaver, and he certainly wanted to live. He started right off by avoiding rigidly his hospital given diet of "bland" cooked foods. He began eating the "forbidden" raw vegetables and fruits, food which he had been warned to leave alone. He drank from 4 to 6 pints of fresh raw vegetable juices every day, 3 or 4 of which were pure carrot juice. He took colonic irrigations and enemas every day for the first 3 or 4 weeks, then tapered off to about 3, then 2 a week. He took daily sun baths lying on green grass—It was April when he first came to see me. As I do not practice I had the Doctor, a Chiropractor, who looked after him for me, keep me posted daily on his progress, and in the following fall, in November, he was able to go to work at his trade. This was nearly 10 years ago. Recently, only a few weeks ago, he walked into my office as hale and hearty as could be, and looking not one day older than he did one year after I first met him. Here was a young man who WANTED to live and to **Become Younger.** By controlling his diet and living habits, with unswerving determination to get well, he has rebuilt his nerve system in a most satisfactory manner.

I have found that injections of every kind, from "shots" to vaccinations and inoculations are very harmful to the nervous system. There is no question about it that they are extremely valuable and beneficial if one wants to develop a speedy means to reach a state of degeneration and premature senility. In this connection, I use the common sense that God placed at my disposal within the cells of my brain, and I discount at least 90% anything I see or hear advertised as "recommended by physicians" or their organizations, particularly when offered free. If we do not pay for it, the City, State or Government does and the manufacturers get their money anyway. In the long run **we** foot the bill. Do not take anything for granted, not even what I say, until you have investigated and put into practice what Nature will do for you. Then, from experience, you will KNOW the TRUTH.

Let us learn to get our nerves completely under OUR OWN control at all times, so we may develop the knowledge and poise so necessary in order to **Become Younger.**

We CAN succeed when we KNOW the Power within us.

Chapter 17.

THE MUSCLES.

The muscles and nerves work in complete coordination and sympathy when the body is healthy and up to par. The nerves furnish the impulses and the motive force, and the muscles carry on the work.

They are so closely related that, often as not, the disfunction of one results in the crippling of the other.

There are many ailments and afflictions which result from the abuse of the muscles, nerves and bones in the body. Most outstanding of all is the abuse which results from the desire to be a victim of fashions. I refer to the wearing of high heels. So disastrous is the damage resulting from wearing high heels that distorted and prolapsed organs and female trouble (in women) becomes more prevalent and pronounced whenever fashion decrees an increase in the height of heels. This damage is rarely discovered immediately. When the trouble begins to be felt, its cause is rarely attributed to the feet, but usually that is where it started. High heels have the tendency to throw every bone, from the foot, the pelvis, the vertebrae, to the region of the brain, out of alignment. This means excessive pressure on nerves, muscles and organs thruout the entire body. I have found that while the natural foot position is as close to the floor or ground as possible, as in walking barefoot, the heel of a shoe should not exceed half an inch in thickness.

Like that of thousands of others, my experience has been that sandals are the most healthy and practical footwear. Feet breathe, they must have as free and unhampered access to air as possible, otherwise toxins and the heavier poisons which gravitate towards the lower extremities are retained in the feet and re-absorbed into the system. This may result in flat feet, athlete's foot and excessive perspiration. I was once bothered with all three of these unpleasant discomforts, but since wearing sandals I have had no foot trouble whatever, not even cold feet. Many shoe stores can supply sandals. Choose the kind and type most comfortable for your feet.

Much of the nerve and muscle trouble which results from lack of proper nourishment may cause the individual to become crippled or lame for life, if not corrected. I have found, for example, that "polio" may be caused by malnutrition on the part of the mother as well as of the victim. The fact that the rest of the world does not yet seem to be ready for this type of science does not discourage me in the least. I have discovered to my own satisfaction the TRUTH as to what succeeds and what fails. Neither I nor my family brook any compromise in our way of living, and I continue my researches day after day to discover everything I can that will lead and help us to **Become Younger.**

I learned years ago that all people are not ready for our diet or mode of living. People choose their food and their pleasures and pastimes according to their state of consciousness. People whose consciousness is extremely physical and material have the mass or herd instinct. Anything that is out of the ordinary, and which is beyond their understanding and comprehension is anathema, idiotic, crazy,—all proof to the contrary notwithstanding.

When a person has risen to a higher state of consciousness, whether by accident or design, he needs food of a higher vibration than the dead cooked and processed foods which include concentrated starches and proteins.

I treasure and value greatly the friendship and appreciation of every one who contacts me to let me know what benefits have been derived from putting my teachings into practice. One of the letters I prized most was one which I received from a lady in Ypsilanti, Michigan, and I would like to share it with you.

It read as follows:

> D . . . was stricken January last year at the age of 2 years old, was PARALYZED, and went BLIND. . . . The Doctors gave him up and said there was nothing they could do for him any more. . . . that the tissues of his eyes were destroyed . . . said they were like an empty shell and there was no hope of his ever seeing again. I heard that CARROT JUICE was good for the eyes . . . Thank the Lord, by Christmas D . . . was seeing again, everybody was amazed over it, and now I recommend CARROT JUICE to everybody I hear suffering . . . Also I want to say D . . . walks around almost recovered.

Another letter is one I received from a Doctor in California, and I quote from it:

> With the Juices I now accept cases that I would not accept without the help that comes from the Juices. Cases of PARALYSIS which are hard at best, respond surprisingly well. . . .

If you were to ask me, again, "Why does not everybody know this?" I would repeat that in the lower state of physical and material consciousness, it would seem, most people would rather take something to give them instant relief and let the future, including the Undertaker, take care of them. They are not foresighted enough to look for the **cause,** and correct IT by a change in the routine of their daily existence.

Muscles have a particular affinity for uric acid. Uric acid is the by-product or end-product of the digestion and breaking down of protein molecules. When one eats meat or any flesh food, the digestive process breaks it down into the fat and amino acid molecules composing it. This process results in the formation of a great deal of uric acid. This acid should be expelled naturally thru the kidneys. In view of the affinity which the muscles have for it, however, they absorb it before it can be expelled. They continue to absorb it until the saturation point has been reached, when in the natural course of events it begins to crystallize. At this point it forms microscopic sharp crystals, which remain imbedded in the muscles. When these muscles are then brought into play by a movement of that part of the body in which they are, these sharp points penetrate the sheathing of the nearest nerves—a warning of trouble ahead. When this happens, we have the first manifestation of trouble which goes by various names. One of these is rheumatism, another is neuritis, and still another, sciatica. There is nothing whatever mysterious about it. It is simply the law of cause and effect coming into manifestation.

I have, over the years, made thousands of Urinalyses, analyses of urine of men, women and children. The normal elimination of uric acid in the case of meat eating people, I found, should be about 35 grams in about 1,000 c. c.(about 1 quart) of urine. The average uric acid content in these analyses was between 3 grams and 5 grams. This means that these people were RETAINING IN THEIR SYSTEM from 7 to nearly 12 times as much uric acid as they should have been eliminating. Most of them were already suffering, or beginning to suffer, from the sharp pains inflicted by the little uric acid crystals piercing the sheathing of the nerves.

It was not surprising to find far too many indications in the urine and the feces of these men and women that premature old age was not too far off. The constant nagging pain of aching muscles helps a lot to streak the smoothness of the skin with little wrinkles which will soon grow into the furrows of the aged.

The most interesting part of these studies and research was to watch the gradual but definite increase of uric acid in regular subsequent monthly analyses, when the people drank a glass of hot water with the juice of a lemon, upon arising, and another at night before retiring. They eliminated all concentrated protein food, particularly meats, from their diet. They drank one or two pints every day of a combination of carrot, beet and cucumber juice made fresh daily. Of course they also omitted all starchy foods.

Naturally, this helped invariably to show a definite improvement with the gradual disappearance of the erstwhile pains and discomforts.

For more than 40 years I experimented with every machine and contraption I could find to extract these juices. I soon discovered that merely to extract the liquid from the vegetable was not enough. The results I obtained were slow and discouraging. It was not until I extracted the juices with the Triturator and Hydraulic Press unit, that I saw results which were as amazing as they were consistent.

To this day we are still using our Triturator and Hydraulic Press in our home. It's an investment, not an expense.

I have a whole stack of Urinalyses before me now, which have been made during the past 20 years, which prove to me beyond question or doubt that the only way to obtain satisfactory and permanent results is by the use of the above method. The Triturator is a scientifically designed grinder which rips open the cells in the fibers of vegetables and fruits, liberating the atoms and molecules of the mineral and chemical elements and the vitamins in these cells. It grinds the vegetables into an exceedingly fine pulp. This pulp is placed in a very powerful hydraulic press which squeezes out the juice and with it these elements and vitamins.

This is the only machine I have found that gives so complete an extraction. Unless the extraction IS complete, the juices are deficient and cannot be expected to give the consistent results I have obtained in my research work. With these juices, people often found their pains vanishing in a surprisingly short time. As their system improved, the wrinkles gradually began to smooth out and they showed every indication that they were on their way to **Become Younger.**

In contrast to these Urinalyses I have mentioned, those which were made for students and others who were eating natural raw foods and drinking their juices, contained the normal average of 15 to 20 grams of uric acid per 1000 c. c. of urine. When one abstains from eating meat, the generation and formation of uric acid takes place in normal quantities and is eliminated thru the kidneys more or less readily. I have not found any habitual raw food consumers, people who have been eating raw foods only, over a period of many years, and have been drinking a sufficient quantity and variety of fresh vegetable juices, who have been suffering rheumatic pains of any kind.

The excessive use of fats, particularly in the nature of fried foods and those cooked in fat, has a very detrimental and degenerating effect on the system and its mobility. Fats form our most valuable reserve supply of energy, just as the storage battery in the automobile has elements in it which enable it to store up the electric current needed to start the engine. Natural fats are contained in small quantities in nearly all vegetables, but they are dissipated and lost when the vegetables are cooked. Avocado or Alligator Pear and olive oil are probably the finest and best quality fat that the body can use.

To keep our muscles young and supple we must feed them the natural foods which contain vital, live, organic elements. These are found in ample quantity in our vegetables and fruits, and are very readily assimilated when we drink our fresh juices.

The idea of developing muscles by means of lifting weights is good only within certain limitations and by the use of judicious exercise that will keep the entire body limber. If we were to concentrate merely on developing bulging muscles of the arms, chest and legs, we would soon find that the muscles in the rest of the body will become unbalanced.

In the development of muscles, diet and rest are just as important as the physical exercise. The matter of breathing is equally important, as the exercise of muscles causes much carbonic acid gas to be formed. This gas is expelled thru the lungs, mostly, and is heavier than air. As we have already explained earlier in this book, it does more harm than good to take in deep breaths without FIRST expelling the heavier air from the lungs. Whenever exercising, therefore, we always go thru breathing exercises which first clean out our lungs of anything that interferes with air reaching the innermost parts of our lungs.

I hope we now have a clear concept of the importance of the care of our muscles while we are struggling to find the safest and surest way to **Become Younger.**

Chapter 18.
THOSE EYES.

If you will study the eyes of those to whom you speak you will see how true it is that the eyes are the mirror of the soul.

You will see eyes that are youthful at any age, and eyes that are prematurely old. You will see eyes that are honest, straightforward and friendly, and those which are crafty, scheming and shifty. You will see eyes that are wondering, dreaming and bewildered, and some which are assured, decisive and dependable. You will see eyes that are happy, joyous and glad, and some that are cheerless, sour and harsh.

As for yourself, study your eyes, because one of the most difficult things in the world is to express a positive soul thru a negative personality, and the eyes express personality.

If your personality is negative, any intelligent person will know it after reading your eyes a few times. On the other hand, when your personality has become positive, by accident or design, magnetism fairly springs out of your soul thru your eyes.

In order to **Become Younger** there is a whole list of endowments which the SOUL must possess, which must manifest thru the eyes. We are really all of us possessed of these endowments, but so many people have suppressed them for so long that they have converted the positive, cheerful, alert and dependable personality of their youthful days into the negative, indecisive one with which they are afflicted today. No wonder they look so much older than their years!

107

If your personality is negative, it means that you do not have the confidence in God and in yourself that is your birthright. You were born as good and fine as anybody. If you have forgotten this fact, of which you had no doubt whatever when you were a child, it means that since then you have not laid a sufficiently firm hand on life, and instead of being in control of life, you have let life get control of you. This is always distinctly visible in a person's eyes.

When we are a positive personality, we are in control of life. It does not mean that we get everything that we want. That, as a matter of fact, might be the worst thing that could happen to us. It does mean, however, that we have learned to balance what we want, as against what comes our way. It means that we have learned to put up with people and conditions which surround us, realizing that nothing is permanent except change. We have learned that only by doing as well as we possibly can, what is nearest at hand, and what happens to be our lot to do, will we be ready for something better eventually.

All these circumstances show very clearly in our eyes, and the manner in which we live and carry out such tasks is indicated in the way in which the soul is mirrored thru the eyes.

I knew a man whose God was money. Of course he would not admit it. In fact he would have been grossly insulted had he been told so. He called it "good business", "taking care of myself", "thrifty" and many other nicknames.

His health failed quite suddenly and he was obliged to retire. His eyes were shrewd. He was honest to the Nth degree and his integrity was absolutely beyond reproach. A Doctor, whom I knew very well, became very friendly with him. By putting him on the proper kind of raw food diet, gradually, but with lots of vegetable juices, he was able to get this man completely on his feet within a matter of 12 or 15 months. One day this man met another man, a very busy one, and they became fast friends. They were now both eating the same kind of raw diet and drinking their juices daily. His new friend was the direct opposite, in the matter of money. He never worried about it, was liberal with his time, money and possessions, so long as he felt he was helping someone. The close association of these two men so completely changed the first one, that his whole personality became almost sublimated. Apart from the fact that his diet had brought back his health and rejuvenated his body, his eyes took on such a magnetic radiance that his whole personality seemed to become glorified.

His greatest trouble was the fact that, being unmarried, nearly every woman he met became infatuated with him. However, he learned that, having reached a higher spiritual plane because of his greater understanding of life, he was now in control of life. These women, on the other hand, living in a state of general frustration, were allowing life to control them. Their eyes showed it as plainly as the nose on their faces.

Of course there is nothing whatever the matter with becoming infatuated with someone. The trouble starts when the infatuation springs from the selfishness which overlooks the value of true friendship and wanders off into the realms of possessiveness. In the higher states of consciousness possessiveness does not enter into any human relationship. On the contrary the greatest happiness is that which we can share with another in perfect and complete understanding of the Universal love which knows no human bounds or bonds. It encompasses every living thing. The more we love those who are closest to us, the greater is our capacity to love the rest of the human race. Conversely, the more we love others, just so much greater is our ability to love those who are closest and dearest to us. There is nothing whatever physical in this Universal love. It is the Love that the Great Master had, with infinite compassion, for every living creature.

I knew a very lovely woman whose inherent capacity to make people happy would have been colossal, if—and a great big IF—she had not been obsessed with jealousy. Her husband was a very fine, upright, home-loving, one-woman man, with a profitable, growing business. Had he been able to read her eyes while he was blinded with love for her, I know he would never in his senses have married her. After two years her jealousy converted her into an unbearably negative woman. He sold his business, left her and went to the other end of the world, supporting her handsomely the while.

The separation, for which of course she alone was entirely responsible, failed to awaken her to the real state of affairs and she became an introvert, her thoughts running wild in a confusion of jealous and frustrated tantrums. Her eyes, which could have been perfectly beautiful, made even those people recoil who wanted her as a friend. Here was the pitiful spectacle of a perfectly lovely soul degenerating into a sour and cheerless personality thru lack of understanding and cooperation.

Learn to be in control of life, so that your soul may sparkle with life's radiance thru your eyes, and show the world that you WILL **Become Younger.**

Chapter 19.
YOUR GLANDS.

The glands of the human body are about as easy for the average man and woman to understand, as the carburetor of an automobile would be to an eskimo woman who had never seen a car. This is due to the faulty system of our education.

As it is, few people know even the location of their glands, and they know less, if anything at all, about their functions.

In order to **Become Younger,** therefore, we MUST BE re-educated, particularly in the matter of these vital little organs. Without this knowledge, it is the easiest thing in the world for the average individual to submit to an operation which may not only be utterly unnecessary, but which may never in this life give him another chance to **Become Younger.**

As a matter of fact, UNLESS we keep our glands young, we ourselves cannot expect to **Become Younger.**

We have in our body a great many glands which we can divide into two general classifications.

In one class we have glands which are like laboratories. They change substances and convert them into other substances different from those first received by them. Other glands in this class act as filters for material going thru them.

In this class we have the liver, the kidneys, the tear glands, etc.

In the other class we have glands which are manufacturing plants. These are known as the glands of

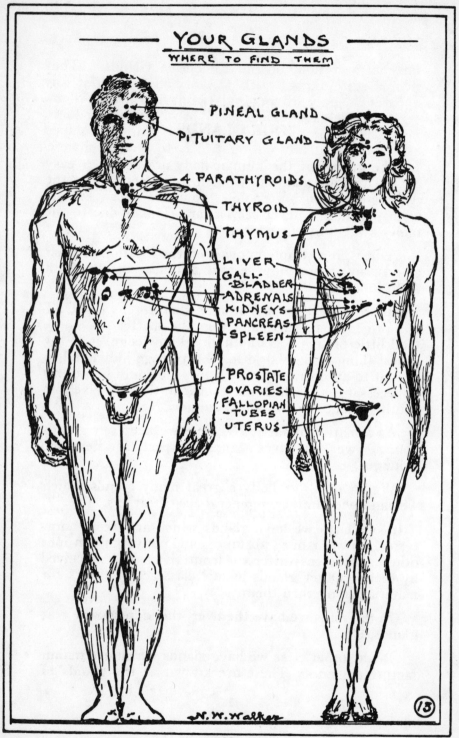

YOUR GLANDS

WHERE TO FIND THEM

PINEAL GLAND
PITUITARY GLAND
4 PARATHYROIDS
THYROID
THYMUS
LIVER
GALL-BLADDER
ADRENALS
KIDNEYS
PANCREAS
SPLEEN
PROSTATE
OVARIES
FALLOPIAN TUBES
UTERUS

N. W. Walker

⑬

internal secretion, or the Endocrine Glands. They manufacture things such as hormones without any apparent supply of materials from outside of themselves. These hormones, and other such products, are secreted or discharged directly into the blood stream without any outlet such as a duct or channel leading from the gland.

We have 8 principal Endocrine Glands, and these are:

Pineal	Thymus
Pituitary	Pancreas
Thyroid	Adrenals
Parathyroids	Sex Glands Group

I have made a large chart of the glands, which I have spent a great many years in developing. It is too large to insert in this book — it measures 17 inches by 22 inches — and as it sells for $5, it would make the price of this book prohibitive to the majority of those who are really interested in its subject, if it were inserted in it.

The chart shows and describes all the principal glands in the body, including the chain of sex glands. It shows the relation and inter-relation of each gland with every other gland. It shows the participation of each gland in the function of other glands. It shows, not only the chemical and mineral elements composing the glands, but also what relationship each of these elements has with other glands. It shows the elements needed to nourish each gland, and the formulas of the vegetable juices which are needed to help each gland to be at its highest efficiency.

As this chart cannot be included here, I have made a sketch for you to study, which will give you a general idea of where the glands are located in the body.

No gland can be said to be more important than any other gland, nor less important. No individual

113

gland is ever afflicted in any manner without at the same time involving, directly or indirectly, every other gland in the system. It is very important to remember this, always.

If a glandular disfunction becomes manifest, and we try to correct it of itself, without at one and the same time balancing the remedy to include some help for the rest of the glands, we may start a chain of reactions which may sooner or later throw our whole system out of order.

In my experience, I have found that it is only in the most extreme case of trouble that we are justified in concentrating on only one or two specific glands, disregarding the others for the time being.

When we study the various glands, the reason becomes apparent.

THE PINEAL GLAND

The Pineal gland is more actively engaged in the business of our "higher" or spiritual self. It is involved, usually in cooperation with the Pituitary gland, in the activities of the brain, such as memory, judgment, reason, contemplation, reflection, love, adoration, pure worship, etc. These activities work along lines of vibrations which are set in motion by the Pineal gland, much like the vibrations of the loud speaker in your radio, only several million times faster.

The activities of the Pineal gland depend upon the spiritual plane on which the individual is living. If he is on the higher spiritual planes, its vibrations have an uplifting emotional influence. If he lives in the lower, material, gross, physical plane the emotions are more in the same class as that of the animals.

I made an interesting experiment along these lines one day. A scientist, friend of mine, developed an extremely sensitive electronic instrument which would register the rates of vibrations from those of the lower animals to those of a highly developed, spiritual individual. I took the "controls" in my hands, while he fingered the dials on his machine. He claimed that a person holding these "controls" could not register any other than his own natural vibrations according to the state of consciousness he was living in at the time. I told him that anyone who had mastery over and control of himself, could raise or lower his vibrations at will. He disagreed with me completely. Hence this experiment.

For nearly a whole hour, I made his indicators jump all over the dials. I caused my pineal gland, at will, to vibrate at whatever rate I wanted. I began with placing myself completely poised, at peace with the world, in a state of ecstasy, on a low stool. I visualized, in a matter of seconds, the life of Christ, and tried to emulate his wonderful love for every living creature. I could literally feel myself sublimated, and I gave my friend the signal to register my vibrations. Imagine his dismay and amazement when the indicator shot way beyond the highest register on his machine.

Next, after a few minutes of "getting down to earth", I began thinking about my French sheep dogs and the litter of pups they presented me with only a short while before. When I gave the signal, the indicator dropped two-thirds of the way down the scale— into the range of animal vibrations.

After a few more minutes, I again concentrated my thoughts, visualizing myself in a hall packed with people watching a prize fight. When I had assumed a sufficient amount of their emotions, I gave the signal, and the indicator dropped to the lower extreme.

This experiment was much more gratifying to me, because it proved to me that I have been able to ob-

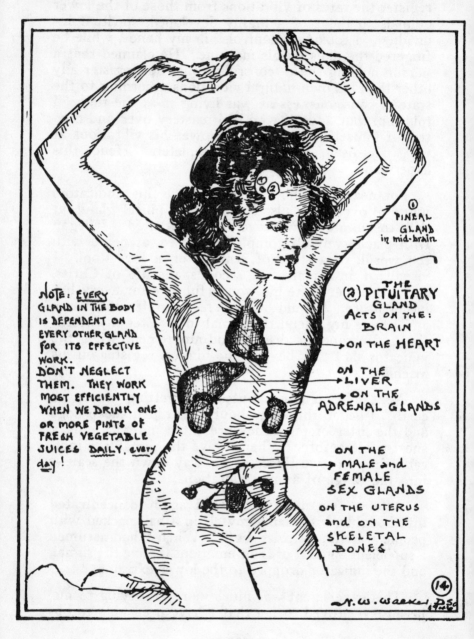

NOTE: EVERY GLAND IN THE BODY IS DEPENDENT ON EVERY OTHER GLAND FOR ITS EFFECTIVE WORK. DON'T NEGLECT THEM. THEY WORK MOST EFFICIENTLY WHEN WE DRINK ONE OR MORE PINTS OF FRESH VEGETABLE JUICES DAILY, every day!

① PINEAL GLAND in mid-brain

② THE PITUITARY GLAND ACTS ON THE: BRAIN
ON THE HEART
ON THE LIVER
ON THE ADRENAL GLANDS
ON THE MALE and FEMALE SEX GLANDS
ON THE UTERUS and ON THE SKELETAL BONES

N. W. Walker D.Sc.

116

tain control over my Pineal gland, and that conse-quently I am in control of life. My friend, however, is still baffled by the result, and is, so far as I know, still wondering how it is done. When he asks me, I will tell him that it is the result of no smoking, no drinking of any alcoholic or "soft" beverage, no eat-ing of meat, grains, starches or sugar, and not letting one negative thought enter my consciousness. It is just as simple as that. But more later.

THE PITUITARY GLAND

The next gland for our consideration is the Pitui-tary gland. It governs the equilibrium or balance of the entire glandular system of the body. If for no other reason, this would be sufficient ground for con-trolling our appetites and training them along the most constructive lines which would lead us to **Become Younger.**

The front part of this gland is concerned with the growth of the body and in the reproductive functions. The hormone which this gland generates serves to stimulate the sex glands.

The posterior, or rear part is involved in the **con-traction** of the muscles, in the pressure of the blood circulating system, and in the color pigment of the skin. It also exerts a controlling influence on the function of the kidneys, **regulating** the passage of water thru them.

The intermediate, or middle part of this gland, on the other hand, exerts a **restraining** influence on the function of the kidneys. Thus we see both functions of the same organ or gland, regulated by different parts of another gland. It is easy to see how the dis-function of the Pituitary gland would cause either an excess or a defect in the flow of urine.

We have found that the starch molecule in grain and flour foods may be blamed for many Pituitary disturbances, disrupting the function of the kidneys. Particularly have I noticed this in the case of bed-wetting by children. When they were taken entirely off cereals, bread and other starchy foods, and given fresh raw vegetable juices instead of milk, this habit of bed-wetting soon ceased. This is not a coincidence, as the difficulty which so many elderly people have in controlling urination may usually also be traced to their copious intake of starchy foods.

Proper nutrition and hygiene for all the cells in our body will enable all the glands to function at their best, without the need of synthetic vitamins and hormones. Only when our glands are functioning at their highest efficiency, will we know that we are really **Becoming Younger.**

THE THYROID GLAND.

The Thyroid is the gland with which most people are familiar, because one of the troubles resulting from its disfunction is the growth of a goiter in the throat. This ailment would not afflict people if they were properly nourished.

The Thyroid has a strong controlling influence on all the chemical processes which are carried on in the body. One of the substances which is created by this gland is the hormone known as "thyroxine". This is the simplified name compounded from the chemicals composing it, namely: trihydro-triiodo-oxyindole- propionic acid. Among the elements or ingredients which the Thyroid uses to make this hormone is a proteid known as **casein.** The body manufactures its own casein out of the atoms present in our food, in the same manner that the cow generates the casein in her milk from her feed. Casein is one of the important components of milk, but when cow's milk is used by humans of any age, it is not digested properly or completely under any circumstances. That is the reason why the use of milk not only creates a great amount of mucus in the system, but also has the tendency to disrupt the function of the Thyroid gland. The casein in cow's milk is 300% more concentrated than that in mother's milk. When cow's milk is pasteurized or cooked by boiling, the casein is changed still worse than in its raw state.

The pasteurization of milk came into being when the large dairies engaged a doctor in one of the Eastern States to have it legalized, so they could distribute milk with less spoilage and consequently at greater profit to them. The claim that such milk prevents the spread of undulant fever is entirely false. As a matter of fact, in my own laboratory I have found that the undulant fever germ will propagate much more rapidly and prolifically in pasteurized than in the raw milk. If you are interested in pursuing this study further, read what I have written on the subject of MILK in my book DIET & SALAD SUGGESTIONS, and see how many deaths resulted directly from the use of pasteurized milk in San Francisco California, and in Montreal, Canada.

From my own observation, I am satisfied with the opinion that youngsters who drink large quantities of milk are building up Thyroid and other glandular troubles in years to come. Fresh raw vegetable juices are far more healthy and nourishing than cow's milk.

When we avoid foods that would be likely to interfere with the functions of our glands, and use, instead those which are constructive and nourishing, such as the raw foods and fresh vegetable juices, we build up not only the resistance of the glands against injury or disfunction, but we enable them to create more and better hormones. In so doing, they enable the entire system to be healthier and more efficient.

119

Unless the Thyroid is able to generate efficiently the thyroxine hormones, many disturbances may result. Among these is the wasting of body tissues, irritability of the nerves, damage to teeth and muscles, affliction of the sex organs, thickening and coarsening of the skin, dry and unsightly hair, to name but a few. These conditions are all regulated by the Thyroid gland and its thyroxine hormones.

In order to **Become Younger,** therefore, we would avoid taking any synthetic or animal hormones, except of course in the most dire extremity as a last resort. The finest and most effective hormones we can get are those which our own glands generate from the proper raw nourishment in our diet.

The effect of the wrong kind of food in our daily diet may be much more serious than a mere passing affliction. It may result not only in goiters, but also in such infirmities as dwarfism (or undersized,) obesity and giantism (or abnormal growth), cretinism or idiocy, and many others. Many of these of course may be the result of mechanical disfunctions of the parts affected, and some may be helped by means of skillful Chiropractic adjustments. Concentrated medicines and drugs may help to correct certain conditions, but only at the expense of damage to the same or other parts of the body at a future date. On the other hand, we have seen remarkable results achieved thru the use of a proper cleansing program, and a properly balanced diet of raw foods supplemented with an abundance of fresh raw vegetable juices properly made with the right kind of equipment.

Unless these juices are properly and completely extracted from the vegetables they are likely to be deficient in the very elements that would be needed for reconstructive purposes. In such a case the results anticipated may be a long time coming. On the other hand I have never yet known it to fail that when the juices were fresh—not canned—and made with the right kind of equipment, they were of definite benefit.

I have in mind the 13 year old son of a New Jersey farmer. When I first met him the little fellow was a typical cretin. His head was oversize, his hair was like dried hay, he had the body of a 5 year old child and was unable to make more than unintelligible sounds thru his distorted mouth. He was brought up almost exclusively on milk and starchy foods.

His diet was completely changed to raw vegetables and fruits, and all the fresh raw vegetable juices he could drink, every day. In the course of 3 years, by the time he was 16 years old, his body had grown considerably and its shape was more normal, his face had acquired a definitely intelligent look, his hair was perfectly natural and vital and he was able to speak like any other member of his family.

Another case was that of a 23 year old girl in California. Up to the age of 14 she had been apparently normal in every respect. Almost overnight her body began to shrink and she lost her ability to speak clearly. In fact her speech was quite unintelligible, except to her family. Her hair became straight and wiry, and her movements indicated plainly a state of idiocy. Her condition did not respond to any of the "orthodox" treatments, and her family finally turned to Natural methods in the hope of getting some benefits for her.

She was given enemas and colonic irrigations. She had been living on starches, milk and canned foods, and it was with some difficulty that she was made to change to nothing whatever except raw fruits and vegetables and of course all the fresh vegetable juices she would drink daily. These were made in their home with a Triturator and Hydraulic Press in order to insure both the quality and the purity of the juices.

A perceptible improvement became noticeable almost immediately, and within a few months her speech could be clearly understood. I last saw her about two and a half or three years after her diet was changed and she was not only quite normal but was resuming studies which had been interrupted when she became afflicted with her ailment.

The juices which were used in both these cases were 2 pints of the Formula #2 in the book RAW VEGETABLE JUICES, What's Missing In Your Body?, consisting of carrot, celery, parsley and spinach to which was added one quarter teaspoon in each pint, of powdered kelp, sea lettuce or dulce which was obtained from the local Health Food Store. In addition one pint of carrot and spinach (Formula #61), one pint of carrot juice and when possible one pint of Formula #30 consisting of carrot, beet and cucumber. This was the daily schedule. When it was impossible to take the 5 pints, then as many as possible were taken in the order given above.

We have known a great many people who used all or most of these formulas to help relieve their goiter troubles, and were greatly benefited as a result.

The Thyroid gland has a lot to do with helping us to rejuvenate, but we must watch what we eat and drink, if we expect it to help us to **Become Younger.**

THE PARATHYROIDS.

The Parathyroids are 4 glands attached to the Thyroid. Their main function is to govern and regulate the calcium supply in the body. They also exert an influence over the lymph system in neutralizing certain types of toxins in the system.

They are responsive to the negative emotions, such as worry, anxiety, fear, anger, hatred, jealousy

122

and so on, under which circumstances they excite or stimulate secretions from the Adrenal glands. As we have already seen, this secretion, Adrenalin, is highly poisonous and affects the whole system when secreted to excess.

The principal function of the Parathyroid glands, however, is the regulation of calcium metabolism, the calcium content of the blood, in tooth and bone formation, and the residual calcium in the tissues. It is most important to realize that these glands do NOT have the SELECTIVE ability to choose between organic and inorganic calcium. That is to say that they will take whatever calcium atoms or molecules come along, irrespective of whether they are dead, or vital, live elements. If our Creator had given them this ability to choose the live and reject the cooked or processed elements, we would have no arthritic victims, we would have marvelous teeth all our lives and no one would have any deformed bones, so long as we ate sufficient raw nourishment.

As it is, the calcium from pasteurized milk and cooked milk products, as well as that from grain and starch foods has become inorganic thru the process of heating. Under these circumstances no matter how much calcium we take into our system by eating these foods or taking calcium in tablet or similar form, the body cannot utilize it constructively without eventual damage to the calcium bearing parts of our system. We have the proof of this in the swollen calcified joints in arthritis, in the degeneration of the teeth and bone, in impactions in our blood vessels as in tumors, hemorrhoids, varicose veins, high and low blood pressure and of course all the signs of premature old age.

In order to **Become Younger** it is necessary to furnish the body with the nourishment rich in **organic** or vital, live calcium elements which the Parathyroids can work with to our best advantage. These elements are found only in the raw vegetables and fruits and their fresh raw juices.

Among the richest calcium foods we have carrots, turnips, spinach, dandelion, to name but a few.

THE THYMUS GLAND.

The Thymus gland is a little known gland whose function changes several times during our life span. In babyhood, up to the age of about 18 months, it breaks down the casein and other elements in the mother's milk, enabling the body to assimilate and utilize the milk or its equivalent. After about 18 months of such work it undergoes functional changes of a remarkable nature. Until puberty and the beginning of adolescence the Thymus gland is involved in the development of the sex glands. With the advent of adolescence it becomes an important factor in the higher and broader expansion of the individual's character and emotions. If the activity of the Thymus in the development of the sex glands has not abated at this time, the individual keeps growing until he is taller than average. On the other hand, if the sex glands develop too soon, and the Thymus is diverted too speedily to the next change in its activity, the individual ceases to grow and remains below average height.

With the advent of adolescence the Thymus acts as a balance between the higher and the lower instincts. It is then controlled by the will, by the mind and by the desires of the individual, until maturity is reached. This period is the most critical in everybody's life. It depends on the extent and severity of the discipline applied to the individual. It is the foundation upon which the future integrity and honesty of the individual is based. If he is allowed to go about his way of life, unbridled, undisciplined and uncontrolled, the

Thymus gland will become flabby in texture and in years to come he will find himself on the lower, if not the lowest, plane of consciousness.

At this period in life the Thymus works in close relation with the Pineal gland, the spiritual gland. When discipline is slack or lacking we find youngsters gravitating toward juvenile delinquency, hoodlumism and crime. Houses of correction and jails are full of such pitiful people, altho it is well to add that there are probably far more people in such institutions who have no rightful business to be in there, than there are outside who should be inside such places.

To develop the character, integrity and honesty of future generations, parents must come to realize that children of all ages NEED affection and understanding, as well the right kind of nourishment. The development of these two highly important character building glands, the Thymus and the Pineal, rests entirely in the hands of parents. When children and adolescents grow into dependable and honorable citizens even tho they were allowed to grow up without guidance, they have done so in spite of lack of discipline and guidance and because of an inherent higher intelligence than that of their parents.

If **we** want to **Become Younger,** we must also give our offspring the opportunity to learn the simple rules that will enable them to **Remain Young.**

THE PANCREAS.

The Pancreas is the most active gland in our digestive system. It produces substances in the form of digestive juices of several different kinds at one and the same time, each to process the various elements contained in the food we eat.

When we eat raw vegetables and fruits, the functions of the Pancreas are at their best. They have virtually no splitting of molecules to do, merely assisting the atoms and molecules to separate so they can be readily collected by the blood and lymph streams and quickly utilized by the glands, cells and tissues thruout the body.

When we eat starches, sugar and meat foods, the Pancreas have to do more than their normal work. Starches cannot be digested as such, but must be converted into primary or chemical sugars. The Pancreas must not only furnish the digestive juices for these sugars but must also help to do the necessary work of conversion or breaking down of the starches. This extra work is what eventually may develop into diabetes.

When we eat meat, fish or fowl, we cannot use either the concentrated protein or the amino acids that compose it, as such. They must all be reduced to the atoms composing them so that the body may reorganize these atoms to build its own amino acids and proteins. The Pancreas does most of this conversion work, furnishing the digestive juices for the purpose. As this task involves considerable work, it not only overworks the Pancreas, but it also generates large quantities of uric acid in the system, as we have already learned in our study of these pages.

Fats contained in the food we eat, must be converted into glycerin, and the Pancreas also furnishes the digestive juices for this purpose.

As the Pancreas has so much work to do for us under even the most favorable circumstances, it is obvious that to overwork it just because we choose to eat food and drink beverages that do actual harm, does not make sense. On the contrary, we should consider this angle of our appetites and desires seriously and with common sense, if we really want to **Become Younger.**

People who insist on giving babies and children candies, cookies and other starchy foods, as well as sugar-sweetened drinks, surely cannot realize what a crime they are committing against the child and against Nature. The horrible and appalling increase in diabetes among children of all ages should surely be a lesson to parents.

To **Become Younger,** in this day and generation, we must use intelligence and common sense. We simply cannot afford to be lured by false and misleading advertising.

THE ADRENAL GLANDS

The Adrenal glands are right on the top of our kidneys, like a cap on each kidney. If you will go back to chapter 8 and read it over again, you will refresh your memory on the potency of the secretion of the Adrenal glands, Adrenalin, and its dire effect on the whole system, both physical and mental. You will recall that one single drop of Adrenalin is diluted instantly to 1 to 2 **billionths** parts of its strength, or one drop of it into 6,000,000 gallons of blood. As the entire body has only about 5 quarts of blood in it, I will leave you to figure out how microscopic is the volume of Adrenalin secreted at one time. Our Creator certainly gave us far more credit than we deserve, when he placed within us such a powerful substance, such a deadly poison.

Death from excessive anger, fright or excitement could readily be caused by too much Adrenalin getting into our blood stream and not being diluted quickly enough. Animals, such as cattle, hogs, etc., herded for slaughter know by instinct their approaching fate. They are filled with helpless fear and terror beyond description. As a result, their blood and muscles become saturated with adrenalin poison. Their poisoned flesh is then immediately attacked by germs. The very moment that life escapes from the body of these animals, their meat begins to decay.

Adrenalin is one of the elements involved in our program of how to **Become Younger.** If we control all our negative emotions, it will give us the necessary stimulus needed for courage, strength and endurance. If we let our emotions go hay-wire, uncontrolled, Adrenalin will help us very quickly to shed our youthfulness and speed up the approach of senility.

If our education had not been sadly neglected when we were tiny tots, and we had been taught all about our anatomy and its functions, we would have learned very early in life that it does not pay to nurse negative emotions. We would have learned very graphically that to give way to anger, to let our bad temper get the better of us, to let jealousy blind us and sway us against all rhyme, reason and common sense, to let worries beset us, and to become the victims of fears of any kind, meant stimulating the Adrenal glands into injecting into our body vast quantities of this insidious, poisonous, concentrated Adrenalin. On the other hand, we would also have learned how the control of all these emotions will help us to the end of our days, to understand, both ourselves and others, to a degree that would make life really worth living.

When the Adrenal glands are healthy and are working efficiently, they inject into the blood just enough Adrenalin for constructive purposes. Under such circumstances, Adrenalin raises the blood pressure, while at the same time it has the opposite effect on the inte - tines, it relaxes them. It **contracts** the capillaries of the blood stream, while at the same time it **dilates** the bronchial tubes. It has such a powerful influence on the heart that, in an emergency, it has been injected directly into the heart of people who have died, within 3 or 4 minutes after the heart had stopped beating, and they were brought back to life. 6 minutes after the heart stops beating, a person is definitely dead.

Adrenalin also dilates the pupils of the eyes and it helps to control the pigment of the skin.

Taking all these functions into consideration, and relating one to the other, we can readily see the chain of events manifesting when we succumb to negative emotions. Anger, worry, fear, jealousy, fright, are all too plainly visible in the dilation of the pupil of the eye, the change in the color of the skin, the rise in blood pressure, to say nothing of the frustration and exhaustion which usually follows.

On the other hand, on the positive side, the Adrenal glands can be, and are, extremely helpful in a great many circumstances. For example, people who have been faced with seeming disaster have been able to perform acts of heroism or self preservation that seemed impossible or superhuman. This was due to the courage instilled into the individual by virtue of the constructive functions of the Adrenals.

I am giving you this information so extensively because self mastery and self discipline are the result of the cooperation we give to our Adrenal glands. This cooperation is one of the most important and vital efforts we must make in order to **Become Younger.**

Take the matter of smoking as another example. The habit of smoking has increased to such a colossal extent during the past 25 years that the production of cigarettes alone has risen by more than 300 BILLION pounds—pounds, not cigarettes—over and above what it was 25 years ago. This increased production has not resulted from the value or benefit of smoking, because smoking has neither value nor benefit for the smoker. Its value and benefit accrues only to the manufacturers, advertisers and the middlemen. This increase is the result of the most insidious, harmful and dangerous advertising propaganda ever developed by the human brain.

As a matter of fact tobacco smoke contains two particularly vicious irritating poisons, nicotine and acrolein. This is carefully omitted in cigarette advertising. Inhaling this smoke stimulates an excessive secretion of adrenalin. It is impossible to smoke, or to be in a room where anyone smokes, without inhaling some smoke. Have you ever noticed how "dopey" people are when they first come out of a smoke filled room?

More than once, when discussing the subject with someone who smokes, I was told: "Oh, smoking isn't harmful; why, my father (or grandfather as the case may have been) smoked all his life and he lived to be 80, 90 and even 100". To this I was obliged to counter: "They lived so long in spite of the fact that they smoked, and not because of it." Smoking is without question a very controversial subject, from the standpoint of the smoker. Nevertheless there are angles to the smoking problem which affect human behavior very adversely.

Smokers do not seem to realize how offensive smoking is to a nonsmoker. They overlook not only the hygienic point of view, but also the fact that one cannot be a tobacco smoker without advertising it to all and sundry by the smell of their breath and the rank odor from their body and clothes. These smells and odors are now-a-days being capitalized by soap and deodorant manufacturers. No amount of washing with soap can destroy the body odor that comes from within the body. Tobacco poisons are collected from the mouth way down to the furthest end of the lungs, by the lymph stream. The lymph, in turn, tries to expel them thru the pores of the skin. Have you ever seen the towels used by a smoker immediately he emerges from a steam bath? They are saturated with perspiration that runs from tan to dark brown in color. It is the nicotine and acrolein which have permeated the body by way of the lymph stream and oozed out by way of the pores of the skin.

Smoking can readily become a habit. It is definitely a very bad habit if you have any consideration for other people. Tobacco smoke is very offensive to those who do not smoke. Have you ever heard a smoker say: "I wish I could quit smoking"? I hear it all the time. Only the other day, a woman we know very well, said to me: "I wish I could quit smoking, but to tell you the truth I really enjoy it." I answered: "That means that you neither wish nor intend to stop. By the way, have you any idea how unwholesome your home smells because of the stale tobacco smoke that clings to the walls and to everything in it? That is why we have not been around to call on you. And also, have you any idea how unclean your breath smells? Even when you have not smoked for some hours, your breath and your body odor are offensive. We like you very much, but none of us can stand these odors, which are repulsive to us." A day or two ago we met her again, more cheerful than we had ever seen her before. She told us she had "quit smoking, forever", that she had burned, in their furnace, a whole carton of cigarettes, and that her husband, who was a non-smoker, seemed to have taken a new lease on life.

Anyone who desires to **Become Younger** and who has any consideration for other people, CAN give up smoking if he wants to badly enough. Don't ever be afraid or ashamed to ask people not to smoke in your office, home or apartment. I will not permit ANY-ONE to smoke in my car, in my home, or on my premises. If they do not like it, I shall be most happy never to see them again. A short while ago I was shopping around for a piece of machinery equipment, the price of which runs into several thousand dollars. A salesman called on me, while I was busy talking to some people who had travelled a long way to see me. I excused myself for a moment and met this salesman. He had just the machine that I wanted, but I sent him away without even giving him an opportunity to present the matter to me. His breath, his clothes and his body reeked of tobacco. He lost a sale which might have netted him several hundred dollars, because of a thoughtless habit.

I want you to understand that I have no objections whatever to anybody smoking, if they want to and they know what they are doing, so long as they do not contaminate the air I choose to breathe. It is their body they are harming and they have just as much right to become speedily aged and senile, as I have to **Become Younger.**

A medical dictionary says: TOBACCO: a heart depressant.

THE SEX GLANDS

The Sex Glands are a group of glands in the abdominal region, which exert a major influence in the physical, mental and spiritual life of the individual. Their influence is so marked that they serve as milestones in dividing the periods of life into childhood, when the glands are in the process of development, maturity, when they have reached the stage of fertility, and old age or senility when their reproductive effectiveness has ceased.

While the division into these periods is purely general, we have to take into consideration the fact that civilized habits have shrunk the effective period of the fertility of man. In this present day, the scale of man's life is entirely distorted because of the general lack of sex education in the home no less than in the school.

Man's procreative ability is limited or shortened because of his eating and living habits on the one hand, and his unbridled incontinence and lack of self control on the other hand. When men and women have learned that continence and self control, together with the avoidance of devitalized foods, can help them to regenerate their bodies and help towards a restoration of vigor and youthfulness, they will have learned an important lesson on how to **Become Younger.**

Merely to **Become Younger** for the purposes of self gratification will do no more than to speed up senility in the natural course of events. It is only when we wish to **Become Younger** for the purpose of living a more useful and intelligent life, that we can truly benefit from the knowledge to be gained in these lessons.

I have the record in front of me now of one of my students of more than 25 years ago. She was in her middle 40's at that time and had just been married for the first time. Her husband was in his late 50's and she looked nearly as old as he did. They were most anxious to have a child, but her old family doctor derided the very idea. She was much too old, he said, to have children, and that if she did become pregnant she would not live thru the ordeal. She took up, and put into practice, this study of Natural principles, and she followed these methods almost religiously. After two years her husband told me she was pregnant and he was very much worried about the outcome. They went thru the ordeal of patient waiting, and in the meantime followed more strictly than ever the diet of fresh raw vegetables and fruits, and an abundance of freshly made vegetable juices daily. She drank not less than 3 pints of carrot juice, a pint of carrot and spinach juice, one of carrot, beet and cucumber, and one of carrot, celery, parsley and spinach juice, daily.

On the allotted day the doctor was present with a surgeon and another doctor, in case of emergency. The woman had very little pain or discomfort and refused to take any anesthetic. When they insisted on giving it to her, it did not have any effect. As the child was born, everything was as comfortable and natural as a birth should be, much to the amazement and consternation of those present.

I saw these parents and their son a few years ago. He was a fine specimen of manhood, brilliant and full of promise. The parents looked not a day older than they did the day they were married. They learned how to **Become Younger.**

The foods which are most harmful to the Sex glands are not only the sugars, the starches and alcoholic beverages, but also the spicy and peppery foods and condiments.

The Sex glands function in close participation with the Pineal, the Pituitary, the Thyroid and the Adrenal glands. All these glands are involved in the production of the "sex-hormones". By the control of the mind and of the emotions these glands are automatically trained to control sex thoughts and impulses in adolescence thru maturity. It is only by training the mind and the emotions thru self discipline that we can develop a thoro understanding and a greater appreciation of the purpose for which we were endowed with these glands.

Will power and self control enable us to convert lustful appetites and desires into noble and worth while aspirations. It makes it possible for us to revert or change the course of the life fluid, which originates from the cerebro-spinal fluid, into the channels of the sublime development of the virtues which we ourselves look for in those whom we admire, honor and esteem.

The Sex glands play a most important part in the program of how to **Become Younger,** and they respond with amazing eagerness to the stimuli of the mind, no less than to the correct food.

Meat of any kind stimulates the sex system in an unwholesome manner. It serves to overstimulate the physical and accentuates the animal nature. I know a man who for years followed quite rigidly a raw food program, and became very much absorbed in the philosophies of the mind and soul in the higher states of consciousness. He was a very virile type of man and as a result of his studies and the practice of what he learned, he became a very highly developed spiritual individual. He met a lady one day and a powerful mutual attraction developed between them. She was a good cook, and before long he slipped into her way of eating, which consisted of the usual run of meat and starches, just as he ate in former years. It did not take long for his higher spiritual nature to become submerged into his animal characteristics. Thereafter he explained his change of views by declaring that man needed meat for vigor. It was only a comparatively short time before this change began to show in his appearance. In the ensuing year or two he lost all the ground he had gained in his energy and vitality and age began to mark him as its victim. Today he looks older than his years, and when I asked him why he did not get back to our way of living he said the lady, who is now his wife, did not approve of raw foods!

It is useless to try to convince people against their will. When they are engrossed in the fleeting pleasures and appetites of this life, without thought or consideration of their effect on the human system, we can only leave them to harvest the results of the seeds they sow. Perhaps some day, when they have suffered enough, they will learn that to **Become**

135

Younger we must forego everything that leads to aging, to senility and to degeneration of the body and mind.

THE LIVER.

The Liver is one of the most important laboratories in our body. Every particle of food we eat, and everything we drink, is broken down into its component parts and carried by the blood to the liver. Here, in its microscopic cells, the atoms and molecules of our food are reconstructed into material which the body uses to replenish, rebuild and repair cells and tissues.

When we eat the raw vegetables and fruits and drink fresh juices daily, the activity of the liver is normal. It then carries on its work of cleansing and construction in a thoroly well regulated manner. The atoms and molecules in their new form and arrangement are sent on their way into the blood stream for distribution to the glands and to all parts of the body. The by-product of this work is not wasted. Together with the used up cells from the blood and from other parts of the system, the liver converts them all into bile. The bile is collected in the gall bladder for storage whence it is used as needed, in many of the activities and functions of our body.

Cooked and processed foods cause the liver to overwork. The atoms and molecules in such foods have become inorganic by virtue of the heat used in cooking and processing. This supply of inorganic or lifeless material is entirely devoid of the magnetism which is needed to assist the body functions in doing their work efficiently. Only live, vital, organic raw food, the vegetables, the fruits, and their juices, can supply elements charged with such magnetism. When these inorganic foods pass thru the liver they interfere with the natural, smooth function of its activity. Besides

136

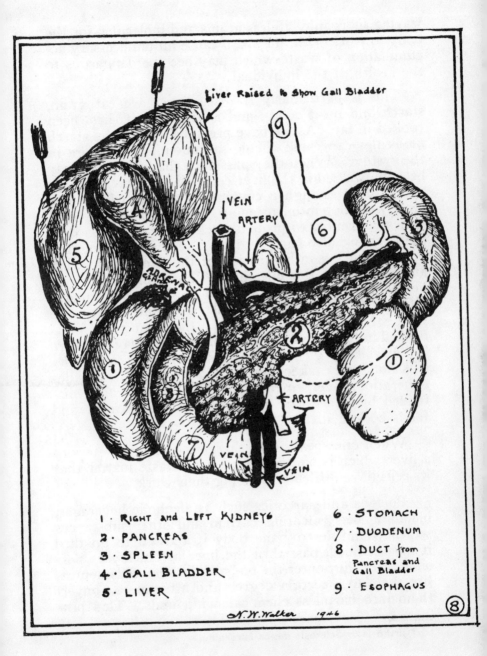

Liver Raised to Show Gall Bladder

VEIN
ARTERY

ADRENAL
GLANDS

ARTERY

VEIN

VEIN

1 · RIGHT and LEFT KIDNEYS
2 · PANCREAS
3 · SPLEEN
4 · GALL BLADDER
5 · LIVER

6 · STOMACH
7 · DUODENUM
8 · DUCT from Pancreas and Gall Bladder
9 · ESOPHAGUS

N. W. Walker   1946

leaving inorganic, lifeless atoms and molecules for the body to work with, they also cause an unnecessary accumulation of waste which may become dangerous to the health of the individual.

This is particularly the case when we eat grain, starch and meat foods, and anything that has been cooked in fat. As we have previously seen, the starch molecules can cause a colossal amount of damage in the system. When they pass thru the liver, they may become wedged in the liver cells. When this has happened often enough a congestion results which may readily develop into hardening or cirrhosis* of the liver. When concentrated protein, such as meat, passes thru the liver, we also run the danger of the cells clogging up and causing inflammation of the liver or clogging and distending the bile ducts. Fat which has been heated to excess, say more than 96° F., is particularly difficult for the liver to handle, as witness the ease with which biliousness follows the eating of foods cooked in fat. No matter how lean meat may be, there is always fat present in it. This is another reason why it is not easily taken care of by the liver. Fatty degeneration, overgrown connective tissue and distended bile ducts are the result of eating meat and foods cooked in fat.

When one speaks of a sluggish liver, one refers to a liver which is so overloaded with waste matter that its cells have difficulty in doing their work.

Poisons and narcotics such as alcoholic beverages, including beer, nicotine, caffein and other substances which would destroy the body if allowed to go thru it uncontrolled, pass thru the liver as quickly as possible after they enter the body. The liver cells neutralize them to a certain degree and attempt to convert them into harmless chemical compounds. This pro-

---

*Cirrhosis or Sclerosis means hardening.

cess, however, involves much more work on the part of the liver than Nature intended for it. It is just like overloading a half-ton truck with about 2 tons of material. Of course the truck will carry it, for a while, but the day of reckoning will involve the expense of a new truck. With our body the circumstances are the same, but the day of reckoning has a different outcome. In the case of the ½ ton truck the tires will give way and the springs will sag, while the frame will become distorted. In the case of man, his feet will lag, notwithstanding, his legs will trail and his body will become bent—in other words he will be old age personified. He will not, however, be able to purchase, acquire or make a new body for himself if he allows himself to get too close to the brink. While there is life, however, there is hope, provided the owner of that life really WANTS to regenerate his body enough to learn how to **Become Younger.**

We have had people come to us who never realized the value of their life until they were so close to the brink that their measurement was all that was needed for the final transaction. It required a superhuman effort for them to change all their habits, but when they did, and when they adhered rigidly to the laws of Nature, they came back to a useful and more intelligent life than they had ever dreamed possible.

One man had graduated from his college with honor and with a swollen head. He was the only one, apparently, who appreciated him and his worth. At 30 he was clerking in a store, at 40 he was doing odd jobs, at 50 he had become a hobo. I gave him a lift on a long and uninhabited stretch of highway in Florida on my way to Miami. His clothes, his body and his breath fairly stunk to high heaven. I thought he was past 60. At the next town he grudgingly accepted my help to get a thoro scrubbing at the Y.M. C.A. and a second hand suit of clothes. When we arrived in Fort Pierce where I had a small grove, I suggested a 3 months' trial of colonic irrigations and raw food and juices, on condition that he work the grove and give up tobacco and alcohol. He accepted, doubtfully, but he carried out his promise and he worked for me for more than a year. When I liquidated my interests there, he continued on my program and with the renewed confidence which followed, he worked himself from one good job into a better one. I met him about 12 or 14 years after. I hardly recognized him. In fact I did not know him, at first; he looked like a man of about 35, full of vim, vigor and health. He was attending a Ministers' convention. Yes, he had become a Minister and was devoting his time and his life to show others, including the down and out hobos, how a man **Can Become Younger,** if he has a mind and the will to do so.

One of the most interesting angles of his "regeneration" is that many times during the first 4 or 5 years of his change of life, doctors and others almost insisted in hospitalizing him because the yellow color of his skin gave definite indications of jaundice. His knowledge of the cleansing processes and functions of the liver made him realize that it was not jaundice, but merely that the waste matter accumulated in his liver was dissolving with the help of the carrot juice and other juices he was drinking daily, and some of it was being eliminated from his system by way of the pores of the skin. When I last saw him he had no trace whatever of any discoloration. On the contrary his complexion was one that any woman might well envy. He was definitely **Becoming Younger.**

THE KIDNEYS.

The kidneys are two organs or glands, each about the size of one's fist. They are suspended in the back, on the rear wall of the abdomen. They hang loosely

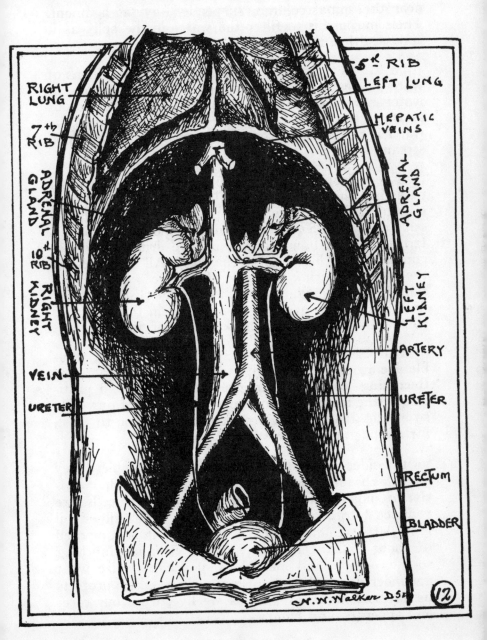

RIGHT
LUNG

7th
RIB

ADRENAL
GLAND

10th
RIB
RIGHT
KIDNEY

VEIN

URETER

5th RIB
LEFT LUNG

HEPATIC
VEINS

ADRENAL
GLAND

LEFT
KIDNEY

ARTERY

URETER

RECTUM

BLADDER

N. W. Walker D.Sc.

12

141

near the spinal column, suspended by a ligament. Their purpose is to filter the water in the body as it is passed thru them by the blood stream.

Small as they are, they filter about 5,500 gallons of water a year. Altho they filter about 4 gallons of water every day, only 2 to 4 pints a day is passed out as waste thru the bladder, as urine. The rest of the water is re-circulated thruout the system, by the blood stream.

Every drop of liquid which enters our system must pass thru the kidneys to be filtered. The blood consists of about 3/5ths water. In other words, 3 quarts out of the total 5 quarts of blood in the body is water. Irrespective of how much liquid we drink, the water content of the blood never changes. All the excess of the water we drink over and above the 3 quarts contained in the blood, is stored in the muscles and in the liver. However, every drop of water in the system is constantly passed thru the kidneys for filtering.

Our Creator very evidently knew how much trouble He would have with us in our efforts to avoid **Becoming Younger.** He made our body, and particularly the most vital and important parts of our body so elastic, that we could continue to live or to exist, for a while at least, in spite of ourselves.

Consider the kidneys as just one example. They are a truly miraculous filtering apparatus. They consist of more than 30 **billion** cells. These cells are grouped into clusters of filter coils. Each filter coil is no larger than a speck of dust, yet it is composed of about 15,000 cells. If you can visualize anything so microscopic and marvelous, you can realize what a wonderful and delicate organ we have which protects us day and night, as long as we live, from our careless appetites and habits.

All drugs and alcoholic beverages are exceedingly harmful to the kidneys, irrespective of the temporary benefits which may be derived by any other part of the body. Beer is probably the most destructive liquid which we can put into our system. I have examined a tremendous number of kidneys at autopsies which I have been able to attend, and I could invariably determine correctly the alcoholic habits of the deceased. I found that beer disintegrated kidneys very fast. In England, where the workingman considers beer and ale his heritage, kidney ailments are the most outstanding afflictions. In the United States, where breweries are on a rampage with their beer advertisements to lure the uninformed and the gullible, kidney ailments are increasing daily. In the brief span of only 10 years, the alcoholic output jumped from less than 350 million gallons, to more than **1 billion 170 million gallons.**

It is only because of the tremendous number of cells in the kidneys, and their miraculous efficiency, that so many people are able to struggle thru a few score years of life, in spite of the destructive liquids which they pour into their system.

"Soft drinks" are nearly always sweetened with sugar. The combination causes alcohol to form in the body, and this must go thru the kidneys for filtering. The damage to children, adolescents and young people, no less than to older people, from the use of such beverages, is almost unbelievable. The insidious part of this damage is that it does not become manifest immediately. It gives a false "up-lift" temporarily, but the subsequent let-down, hours or days afterwards, is rarely if ever attributed to the use of these beverages.

The water in the human system is one element whose importance surpasses that of all the other elements, except oxygen in the air.

Youthfulness in man and woman is determined mainly by the fluidity of its vitality. Vitality must flow constantly and freely thru the entire system. This vitality is dependent on the purity and fluidity of the blood stream and the lymph which in their very nature hinges on the **quality** of the water in the body.

Water that is not constantly replenished becomes stagnant and polluted. In the body, such stagnation results in sickness and disease and is manifested as body odor, or a pale, sallow or ashen complexion. This means premature aging.

The abundant use of fresh raw vegetable and fruit juices furnish the body with the very finest quality of **organic** water obtainable. If we drink enough of these juices, we need hardly ever drink any water. I personally do not drink a glass of water a year except the hot water and lemon juice which I drink every morning upon arising. BUT I drink as much of the fresh vegetable and fruit juices as I can conveniently take. I find that the lemon juice in hot water helps wonderfully to flush the liver and the kidneys. On the other hand I have found that by drinking it cold it helps to stimulate the peristalsis of the intestines and frequently helps the early morning elimination.

Have you ever wondered why so many liver and kidney pills are advertised so extensively? It is because it is a known fact that liver and kidney troubles and ailments. are on the increase. The reason is the increased consumption of beverages and foods which damage these organs, on the one hand, and on the other hand, insufficient education on the value and benefits of the fresh raw vegetable juices.

May I suggest, as good educational reading on the subject, that you obtain a copy of the book RAW VEGETABLE JUICES, What's Missing In Your Body?

A lifetime of study and research has gone into compiling it. You will find listed in it the juices most beneficial and helpful, and the best way to extract them. Innumerable people have written to me saying that this book has been a means to help them rejuvenate, to **Become Younger.**

Chapter 20.

CONSTIPATION

The pace of modern living is responsible for the most prolific ailment of the present day, namely: premature old age.

Constipation is undoubtedly the most important contributing factor in the premature aging of men and women.

There are two crimes against Nature which present day civilization indulges in as a daily routine, which beget this, the most common and popular of our ailments, constipation. One is neglecting to NOURISH the organs responsible for the evacuation or elimination of waste matter. The other is neglecting to stop everything we are doing when the urge to evacuate the bowels should drive us headlong into the bathroom.

Very few people understand what takes place after the food has gone thru the stomach and small intestines, and reaches the lower intestine or the colon. Parents are criminally negligent when they fail, from their own lack of knowledge (which is no excuse), to teach children why their prompt attention to bowel evacuation is extremely important.

Again I want to emphasize the negligence of teachers and of the Boards of Education in failing to teach children anatomy and the functions of the human body. See how long YOU have had to exist before you realized and appreciated the value of this vital knowledge. Think for a moment how far you yourself will have to retrace your steps in order to get **Natural** elimination and a normal colon.

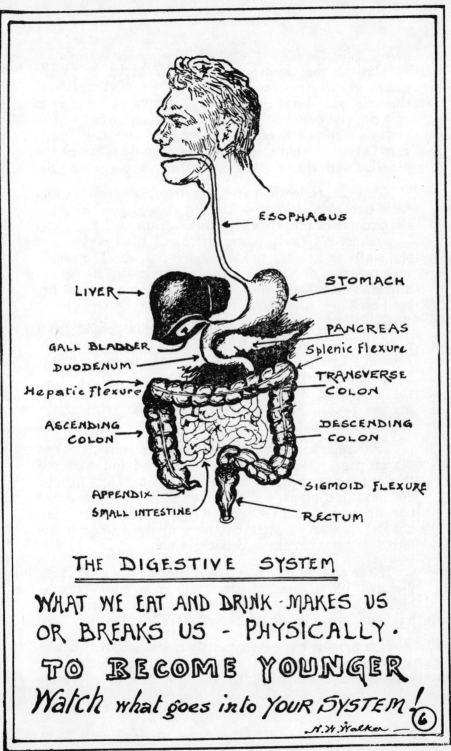

ESOPHAGUS

LIVER →

STOMACH

GALL BLADDER

PANCREAS

DUODENUM

Splenic Flexure

Hepatic Flexure

TRANSVERSE COLON

ASCENDING COLON

DESCENDING COLON

APPENDIX

SIGMOID FLEXURE

SMALL INTESTINE

RECTUM

THE DIGESTIVE SYSTEM

WHAT WE EAT AND DRINK MAKES US
OR BREAKS US - PHYSICALLY.

TO BECOME YOUNGER

Watch what goes into YOUR SYSTEM!

⑥

N. W. Walker

Out of the thousands of X-ray pictures of the colons of different people, men, women AND children, the only ones I have ever seen that approach the lines of a normal colon have been those of children born of women who practiced our program of diet and cleansings before the children were born, and continued the practice with the children while they were growing up.

You can collect a vast amount of information and facts over a period of 40 or 50 years, if you pursue a research with diligence and perseverance. I have collected more X-ray pictures of colons than would line the walls and ceilings of a sizeable house. The recurrent outlines of various parts of the colon in relative ailments has been one of the most amazing of my studies.

I have made a sketch of what would be considered a more or less normal outline of a truly healthy colon. I would like to have you study this very carefully. Note particularly the names of the various parts of the anatomy, of the glands and of ailments, with arrows pointing to the general location with which these are related.

Now turn to the next picture of the colon, marked 10, on page 150 and see how devitalized and distorted this one is compared to the normal colon. Now turn to the next one, on page 151 marked 11 on the right hand bottom corner, and see what happens more often than not, when waste matter has been allowed to accumulate for years, in the ascending colon.

If for any reason you doubt the accuracy of these pictures, I would suggest that you go to some reputable and dependable Chiropractor or Naturopath and have an X-ray made of YOUR OWN colon.

If a person has eaten mostly cooked foods, living on the type of food that is served in most homes and restaurants, his colon cannot possibly be efficient, even

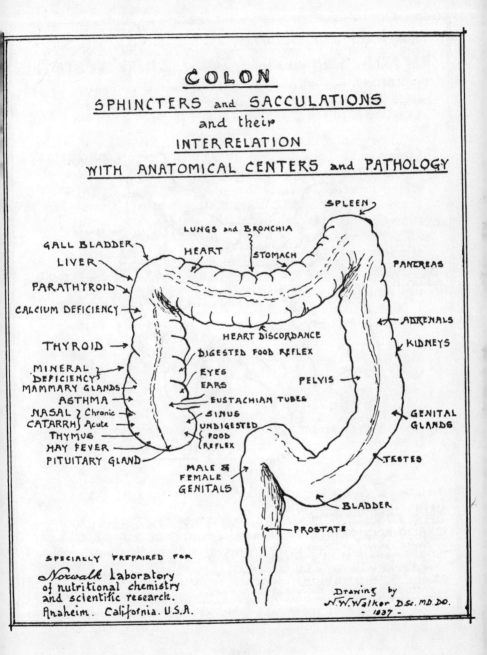

COLON

SPHINCTERS and SACCULATIONS
and their
INTERRELATION
WITH ANATOMICAL CENTERS and PATHOLOGY

SPLEEN

LUNGS and BRONCHIA

GALL BLADDER

HEART

STOMACH

LIVER

PANCREAS

PARATHYROID

CALCIUM DEFICIENCY

ADRENALS

KIDNEYS

HEART DISCORDANCE

THYROID

DIGESTED FOOD REFLEX

MINERAL DEFICIENCY

EYES

MAMMARY GLANDS

EARS

PELVIS

ASTHMA

EUSTACHIAN TUBES

NASAL Chronic

CATARRH Acute

SINUS

GENITAL GLANDS

THYMUS

UNDIGESTED FOOD REFLEX

HAY FEVER

PITUITARY GLAND

TESTES

MALE & FEMALE GENITALS

BLADDER

PROSTATE

SPECIALLY PREPAIRED FOR

Norwalk laboratory
of nutritional chemistry
and scientific research.
Anaheim. California. U.S.A.

Drawing by
N.W. Walker DSc. MD. DO.
- 1937 -

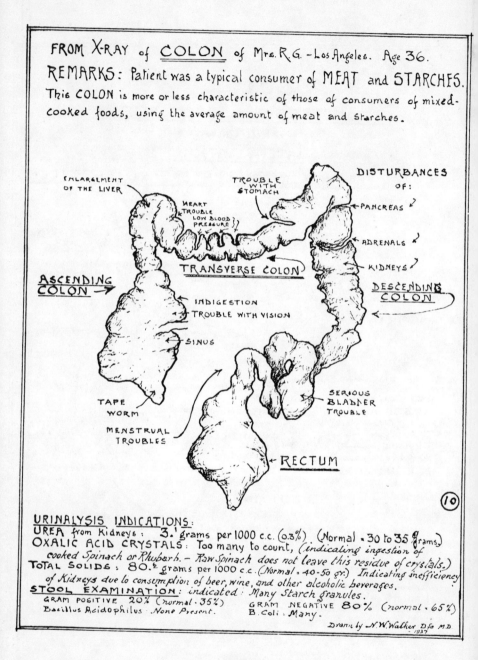

FROM X-RAY of <u>COLON</u> of Mrs. R.G. - Los Angeles. Age 36.

REMARKS: Patient was a typical consumer of MEAT and STARCHES. This COLON is more or less characteristic of those of consumers of mixed-cooked foods, using the average amount of meat and starches.

ENLARGEMENT OF THE LIVER

TROUBLE WITH STOMACH

DISTURBANCES OF:

HEART TROUBLE LOW BLOOD PRESSURE

PANCREAS

ADRENALS

KIDNEYS

TRANSVERSE COLON

<u>ASCENDING COLON</u>

<u>DESCENDING COLON</u>

INDIGESTION
TROUBLE WITH VISION

SINUS

TAPE WORM

MENSTRUAL TROUBLES

SERIOUS BLADDER TROUBLE

<u>RECTUM</u>

(10)

<u>URINALYSIS INDICATIONS</u>:

UREA from Kidneys: 3.¹ grams per 1000 c.c. (0.3%) (Normal = 30 to 35 grams)

OXALIC ACID CRYSTALS: Too many to count, (indicating ingestion of cooked Spinach or Rhubarb. - Raw Spinach does not leave this residue of crystals.)

TOTAL SOLIDS: 80.² grams per 1000 c.c. (Normal = 40-50 gr.) Indicating inefficiency of Kidneys due to consumption of beer, wine, and other alcoholic beverages.

STOOL EXAMINATION: indicated: Many Starch granules.

GRAM POSITIVE 20% (normal = 35%)   GRAM NEGATIVE 80% (normal = 65%)
Bacillus Acidophilus = None Present.   B. Coli = Many.

Drawn by N.W. Walker D.Sc M.D.
1937

150

TRANSVERSE COLON

← ASCENDING COLON
CUT and OPENED
HERE to show SMALL
HOLE in center of
INCRUSTED HARD
FECAL MATTER MORE
THAN 20 years IN
COLON !!!

DESCENDING COLON

↗ From
SMALL
INTESTINE

Appendix   ←RECTUM

The lady whose X-ray picture is copied above, thought her colon was alright, that she was NOT constipated, because she had 3 "regular movements" nearly every day.

Actually, this COLON is in a very serious condition — Look at the solid impaction at the cross-section, where the ascending colon has been divided, showing only a ~ small hole in center of thick black wall.   The - accumulation of more than 20 years !!   The result of eating too much cooked food ~ particularly :- starchy food : bread, cereals, cake, &c.

The entire colon shows plainly a desperate lack of VITAL FOOD.

TO BECOME YOUNGER THE COLON MUST BE CLEAN - HEALTHY - and NOURISHED WITH LIVE, VITAL FOOD.   Carrot-and-Spinach Juice, fresh, raw, is the finest organic nourishment for it.

N. W. Walker 1936

⑪

tho he may have a bowel movement 2 or 3 times a day. Instead of furnishing nourishment to the nerves and muscles, cells and tissues of the walls of the colon, cooked foods actually cause starvation of the colon. A starved colon may let a lot of fecal matter pass thru it, but it is unable to carry on the last of the digestive and nourishing processes and functions intended for it.

The bulk which is so essential for the proper and complete digestion of our food, is needed in the colon just as much as in the small intestine. Such bulk, however, MUST be composed of the fibers or roughage of the RAW foods. When these fibers pass thru the intestines they become, figuratively speaking, highly magnetized and in this condition are very helpful in the peristaltic, or wave-like motions of the intestines, as well as in the processes and functions involved in the various parts of the intestines.

When food is cooked, however, these fibers become completely demagnetized and in this state pass thru the system with little or no benefit. Eventually, experience has proved, these foods leave a coating of slime on the inner walls of the colon like plaster on the wall. In the course of time this coating may gradually increase its thickness until there is only a small hole thru the center. When this occurs, the victim may be totally unaware of it, and go happily having copious passages of feces one, two or three times a day. He does not know that he is actually chronically constipated, as the matter so evacuated may contain much undigested food from which he derives little or no benefit. Sooner or later his collapse is virtually certain, and he may die happily in the illusion that his elimination was "regular," not realizing that the contributing factor to his demise was actually chronic constipation.

The better known constipation is that which manifests as the slowing down or actual stoppage of bowel movements. This particular type is so common that billions of dollars' worth of laxatives and cathartics are advertised in print and on the air every day of our lives. Only the other day a chain drug store ran at a tremendous expense a full page advertisement in the Los Angeles papers advertising a laxative under the heading: HOW TO LEARN TO LIVE AGAIN. Undoubtedly this colossal expense was incurred in many other cities, because people who are constipated usually do not want to do any thinking for themselves and will flit from one remedy to the next with the fervent hope they will not have to resort to dynamite or some other explosive in the end.

The laxative and analogous trades have skillfully spread propaganda to the effect that enemas and colonic irrigations are harmful for some fantastic reason or another, and that they are habit forming. This as a matter of proven fact, is utterly false. On the other hand we have found without exception that the use of laxatives and cathartics is not only habit forming, but decidedly destructive to the membrane of the intestines.

If waste matter has accumulated in the colon, and the bowel does not expel it in a natural manner, it means one of two things: the passage is thoroly clogged up, or the membrane or walls are so flaccid, feeble and impotent that loops may have formed or the channel may have doubled up on itself, preventing the free passage of the feces.

What happens when a laxative appears in the colon? It does NOT cause a resumption of the peristalsis. It irritates the nerves and muscles in the colon. These are lashed into a convulsion which attempts to expel the irritant and in doing so of course some of the feces is expelled with it. If the peristaltic function is missing, failing or dormant, only an irritant would cause such a convulsion in the colon. Therefore

153

I would not expect to find any laxative which is not an irritant, any claims to the contrary notwithstanding.

If I had seen only a few colonic irrigations give successful results, I would be justified in withholding my judgment in regard to their efficacy. Having seen literally thousands of them, all giving results which no laxative or cathartic could give, I must admit that I am dumbfounded whenever ANYONE questions their value or efficacy. As a matter of fact long ago I arrived at the conclusion that no treatment of any ailment, sickness or disease could be effective unless and until the waste matter had been washed out of the colon by means of colonic irrigations, if available, or high enemas if they were not available.

Of course there is a great difference between colonic systems and their operation. The operator should be a person trained in anatomy and particularly in the irregularities likely to be encountered in the infinite varieties of colons. I have found that no inorganic material whatever should be placed in the water. If anything were needed I would use the strained juice of lemons, for example, which helps to neutralize the excessive acidity likely to be present in the fecal impactions in the colon.

There is a difference between the excessive acidity of the contents of the colon and the acid-alkaline ratio throughout the system. Dr. D. C. Jarvis, M.D., has done invaluable research on this subject which, in conjunction with fresh raw vegetable juices, I have found to be of inestimable value in gaining and maintaining a maximum of health and energy. He recommends, and I have found very beneficial, the daily use of a combination of 2 teaspoonfuls of apple cider vinegar and 2 teaspoonfuls of honey in a glass of water. Get Dr. Jarvis' book ARTHRITIS AND FOLK MEDICINE and study particularly this subject on pages 78 and 79 (Edition of 1960). ALSO read the chapter on VINEGAR in my book RAW VEGETABLE JUICES, What's Missing In Your Body?, the Revised, Enlarged 1970 Edition.

Now back to colon irrigations.

It takes an average of from three quarters of an hour to a whole hour to give a good colonic. Almost any machine will do the work well enough, always provided of course that the operator is efficient.

I have found that an X-ray picture of the colon is an invaluable aid to the operator. With it one can work intelligently, as it gives the key to the kind and type of treatment which will be most effective. Furthermore, having studied the X-ray picture and compared it to the "normal" colon which I have sketched in this chapter, you can yourself figure out what the most important disfunctions are which have to be corrected.

In studying your X-ray picture you may find it to contain some fantastic contortions. Don't become alarmed by them. Pretty nearly everybody has them. Just study them from the point of view that it has taken all these years for it to get into that shape and condition. You cannot therefore expect to correct it in 24 hours, or even in one year. Realize that you intend to **Become Younger,** that you have to work long and hard to achieve that goal, and that the straightening out and correcting the condition of your colon will help you every bit as much as going on the right diet and drinking your vegetable juices.

It would take volumes to go completely into the subject of constipation, its cause and how to remedy it. I do not have the space here at my disposal to do complete justice to this vital and extremely important subject. However there are many angles that must be covered, even tho I may do no more than touch the high spots.

One can NEVER be sure that one is not constipated, even when one seems to have several bowel movements daily. I would like to give you the record which I have here before me, of a young woman in her late 20's. She had suffered epileptic fits regularly every month, since her menstrual periods began when she was about 13 years old. No orthodox treatment helped, and no hospital or therapeutic clinic gave the slightest relief. Her family brought her to meet me and I advised taking her to a Nature Doctor for a series of colonic irrigations. It was suggested that she take a colonic every day, 6 days a week, for 5 or 6 weeks. Her family objected, at first, on the ground that the young lady was not constipated but on the contrary was exceedingly regular in her evacuations. When an X-ray of her colon was made, however, for the first time in her life, I could see many disturbances, not the least of which was every indication that there were worms present. She began taking colonics. Each day there appeared thru the colonic glass indicator tube little more than some feces and some strings of mucus, until, after the second or third week her father and the rest of the family began to suspect there was nothing to this system except the money he was paying out. I convinced him that the colonics should continue for the agreed period and he consented. One day, during the 5th week, the young woman sat suddenly upright on the table and in a minute or two passed a mass of worms as large as my fist. During the next few days a few more worms passed out and she began to feel—as she put it—that she had been lifted "out of the depths". The daily colonics were then discontinued, but she took one every week thereafter for several weeks.

Her epileptic fits vanished completely with the expulsion of the worms, and when I saw her again a year or two ago, 10 or 12 years since I first met her, there had been no recurrence of her trouble, and she looked not one day older than the first time I saw her. Naturally, thruout all that time, she had followed my program of a raw diet and vegetable juices.

Another instance is that of a young man who was discharged from the army. Before induction his bowels moved regularly and he had more strength and energy than he knew what to do with. After the injections and inoculations he received under the army medical regulations, his bowel movement became very irregular and he gradually lost energy and ambition. He lost weight, notwithstanding the fact that he developed a voracious, gluttonous appetite which he seemed unable to satisfy. He took a series of colonic irrigations, after the X-ray picture of his colon was explained to him. He took one daily, and at the end of 3 weeks he passed a huge tape-worm and a mass of smaller ones. For about a week thereafter he was very much nauseated, but the judicious use of vegetable and fruit juices soon brought back his appetite, and with it he regained much strength and energy.

One of the dangers of letting waste matter accumulate in the colon, is the absorption, principally while we sleep, of poisons which are generated as a result of putrefaction. Carbolic acid is one and Indol is another. These two are probably the most serious, as they result in headaches and lassitude, to begin with, and may eventually develop into biliousness, paralysis of the intestines and peritonitis. A deficiency of hydrochloric acid secretion in the digestive system is also a condition resulting from the presence of indol. You can readily understand why these conditions respond so readily to colonic irrigations as part of the treatment to remedy them.

The function of the colon is not merely to expel waste matter from the system. The first part, or ascending colon, must absorb all the liquid and the elements which the small intestine failed or was unable to collect. For this purpose it mulches the material which passes into it from the small intestine, and transfers the liquid and other elements thru its walls into the blood stream. By the time the residue reaches the Hepatic flexure, or the uppermost part of the ascending colon, it becomes somewhat more dense, and passes into the transverse colon. With a little more similar treatment here it finally becomes feces and is ready for evacuation thru the descending colon.

Once the walls of the ascending colon become plastered with slime, they very obviously cannot carry on the final processing of the food we eat. The consequent result is a starvation of which we are not conscious but which causes old age and senility to race towards us with the throttle wide open.

An impacted ascending colon is therefore a definite cause of constipation. But it can also and at the same time become the cause of chronic diarrhea. This sounds like a contradiction in terms, but let me give you just one of several instances which have come under my direct notice.

It is the case of a woman who had been afflicted with very severe diarrhea for 6 or 7 years, without any relief. She was also troubled with inability to urinate. Much too frequently she would have the urge to urinate, but could discharge no more than a few drops at a time. She submitted to drugs, medicines and injections any time she was told she could obtain relief but to no avail. She had been given enough "shots" to kill a rhinocerous, and every one made her more sick than ever.

She consulted a doctor friend of mine who asked me to give him my opinion. I thought, by her looks, that she must be about 55 or 60 years old, but her "case card" gave her age as 42. As soon as I saw her I told my friend that if I were in his place I would immediately start giving her colonic irrigations. Both he and his patient laughed at the very thought of such procedure. However, we took an X-ray picture, which confirmed my suspicion, and he finally agreed to try some colonics, altho still declaring that a colonic was intended for a stoppage of the bowel and not for such a copious running-off.

In less than 6 colonics she expelled some 15 pounds of stale fecal matter. Her diarrhea then gradually ceased and the removal of the fecal impactions which were crowding the colon against the bladder enabled the passage of the urine to become normal.

Needless to say most of the strain which made her face look so old, disappeared, and before long she was looking more like a 42 year old.

I never lose an opportunity to emphasize the fact that unless we KNOW definitely, what the condition of our colon is, as indicated in the outline of two or more X-ray pictures, we cannot afford to deceive ourselves into "thinking" that it is alright. Several bowel movements a day are not a sufficient indication that all is well, if we are eating foods that are cooked or processed. Even on a rigid program such as mine, we cannot afford to overlook the possibility that elimination of waste may not be perfect. We are living at too fast a tempo to gamble on wishful thinking. The very speed of present day existence, with all the concomitant civilized problems, conspires to age us prematurely. We must therefore constantly watch ourselves, if we would **Become Younger.**

Not the least of our troubles in connection with the condition of our colon is the generation of gas. Here again we are hemmed in by conventions and proprieties which cause us to retain and reabsorb toxic gases which should be expelled the moment we have the urge to do so. Of course when people are around us this is neither possible nor gracious. However, the use of high enemas has been very helpful to reduce the development of gas.

By observation we can often learn which foods create more gas than others and by avoiding them for a while gas can often be reduced to a minimum.

You may be interested in the case of a little lady whose age I would judge to be about 50, altho she may not have been any older than 40. I never asked her age, but she had a son who was 18 years old. She was having a great deal of trouble in the abdominal region. She would bloat until it would seem that the skin would break. The doctors she went to wanted to "tap" her to remove what they thought was water. She had one movement of the bowel regularly—every other day. No one had ever told her to take enemas or colonic irrigations. She was extremely nervous and was constantly on the border of hysteria. Urged to take daily colonics for a week or two, she passed pint after pint of solid, hard, foul smelling feces which gave every indication of having been stored in her system 20 years or more. I examined some of these particles under the miscroscope and counted millions of gas forming bacteria. During the two first weeks of her colonics she expelled vast volumes of gas in addition to more than 2 gallons of this hard, stale fecal matter.

I am thoroly convinced that the greatest friend of a constipated colon is starchy food. Starches are the most prolific media for the propagation of gas forming bacteria. If I wanted to generate great volumes of gas in my system I would start with some toast, (white whole wheat, soy or any other kind) or hot cakes for breakfast, donuts and coffee for lunch, and noodles, spaghetti, cake etc, for dinner. I know I would also become beautifully constipated on such food. Furthermore I know perfectly well that on such food I would never expect to **Become Younger.**

At one of my lectures a little old lady heard me hold forth against starches, toast and everything of the kind. During the question period she stood up and proudly said: "I toast my bread in the oven until it is thoroly dry and hard. Isn't that much better". I answered: "My dear lady, neither one is good for you; however if you make toast out of your bread, when you throw it out of your window it will go much farther than the slice of bread would."

Bread is already a dead, lifeless food. To toast it, ever so thoroly, just helps to make it still more dead. To speed up the approach of old age, use dead, lifeless food.

To **Become Younger,** however, eat food that is raw, vital and nourishing.

There is quite an important difference between an enema and a colonic irrigation. It is virtually impossible to wash out the colon completely by means of an enema. A colonic on the other hand is administered while the patient is lying more or less relaxed on the table or cabinet while the operator does all the work. The average individual enema uses about 2 quarts of water. When this has been injected and expelled, of course one can refill it as often as wanted or as needed. This involves getting up, sitting down and moving around, all of which under the circumstances is quite beneficial. A colonic enables the operator to inject just as much water at a time as is necessary to wash out each part of the colon in turn, letting the water be expelled and more injected without any effort on the part of the patient. In this manner the operator can use many gallons of water, injecting of course only a quart or two at one time, in one continuous treatment for three quarters of an hour to one whole hour.

In the enema, the temperature of the water is unchanged during each fill or refill of the container, whereas in the colonic the operator can control the temperature at will for any part of the treatment, thus obaining results which only a change in the temperature of the water can give.

However, I consider an enema outfit even more important than a tooth brush, whether at home or while traveling. Also there are many times when a colonic is neither practical nor possible to obtain, and an enema will help at all times. If you wish to form in your mind an idea of the value of enemas, just look at or listen to the advertising of remedies for headache, fatigue, backache and instead of the fizzy product, tablet or pill advertised for the purpose, substitute enemas. You will then have a Natural remedy to help the situation, instead of something that is guaranteed to dull, numb or deaden the nerves temporarily, with subsequent troubles not mentioned.

In extreme cases any remedial substance may be better than a period of agony, but even in such circumstances I have found enemas invaluable.

In taking an enema I have found that the most effective method is to use a medium size, soft pliable rectal tube, about as large around as a lead pencil, size No. 22, 30 inches in length, instead of the short hard black rubber tube. This makes it possible to have the clear water enter past the rectum and lower end of the descending colon.

The enema bag or can should contain about 2 quarts of tepid water, neither hot nor cold, into which the strained juice of 2 lemons is added. The bag, or can, should be hung at a convenient height to permit the water to flow freely. Some people prefer to have it as high as possible so that the flow of water is more pronounced, while others prefer to have it 3 or 4 feet above the ground. A little practice will soon determine which is the most comfortable. The rectal tube, which will previously have been connected to the end of the long rubber tube from the bag or can, with a glass connecting tube or the hard rubber tip, should be lubricated with a vegetable lubricant, such as KY jelly which can be obtained at almost any drug store before preparing to take the enema. Just enough should be squeezed against the rectal tube to lubricate it all the way around and the whole length of it. It will also help

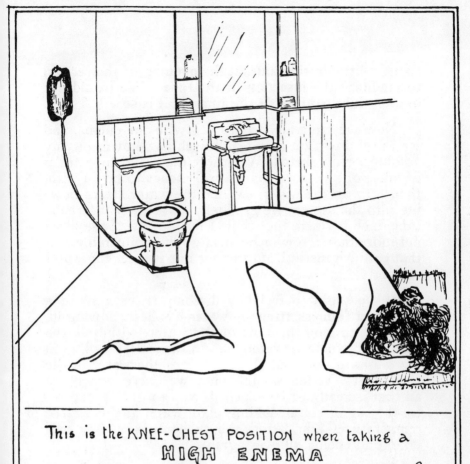

This is the KNEE-CHEST POSITION when taking a
HIGH ENEMA

Use a 30 inch thin Rectal Tube so the water will flow directly way inside the Colon.

The KNEE-CHEST position helps the water to flow in by gravity into the Transverse and Ascending Colons as it leaves the Rectal Tube. It will thus reach the farthest parts of the Colon with less effort and greater efficiency.

It is much more beneficial to use the juice of 1, 2, or 3 lemons in 2 quarts of water, than to use *any-thing* else. We *never* use soap, salt, bicarbonate of soda, &c. We use only lemon and water, or just plain water, neither hot nor cold_ just comfortably tepid. To lubricate the tube we use K-Y jelly.

To BECOME YOUNGER keep the Colon CLEAN !!

N.W.Walker.

(17)

to use a little in the anus, at the opening of the rectum to facilitate the insertion of the tube. We would not use any lubricant made of mineral oil base.

Now we are ready to proceed with the enema, and we kneel down on a rug or towel, as shown on my accompanying sketch. We insert the rectal tube for a distance of not more than 2 or 3 inches to begin with, then turn on the water. While the water starts flowing into the system we gradually and slowly insert the tube, inch by inch, the whole length of it. Sometimes not more than a few inches will go in comfortably. In that case we insert it no further but just let the water run in.

If we begin to feel any discomfort, cramps, or a feeling of fullness after the water has been flowing in, it is best to stop the flow of the water, withdraw the tube, and expel the water, etc., in the toilet bowl, even tho we have not used all or much of the water in the bag or can. When we feel that we have evacuated all that is ready to be expelled, we can get up and re-fill the bag or can by adding plain water at the desired temperature, lubricating the tube once more, and taking an enema all over again.

A little practice by taking a few enemas as and when needed or desired will soon teach us the most satisfactory procedure for our individual case. I consider the use of enemas extremely important in our efforts to ward off old age and in our program to **Become Younger.**

It is a good practice to remember to clean both the bag and the tube with warm water and soap, and thoroly rinse them with cold water before putting them away.

Chapter 21.

JUICES and JUICERS.

You cannot help but be impressed seriously by my stressing the importance of internal cleanliness by means of enemas and colonic irrigations instead of by the use of laxatives and cathartics.

The use of fresh raw vegetable juices is absolutely as essential, in my experience, as enemas and colonics. They are exactly on a par in relation to their importance.

The two vital, cardinal reasons for using vegetable juices is to obtain the finest and best organic water from the vegetables, and to extract from the vegetables and collect in that organic water all the organic chemical and mineral elements and vitamins which it is humanly and mechanically possible to obtain.

This problem confronted me when I first made my careful investigation into the effectiveness of the various juices and combinations of juices in connection with the many ailments I was trying to overcome.

I began, more than 40 years ago, by passing the vegetables thru a meat grinder. I collected some juice in this manner, but soon discovered that the process caused the pulp and the juice that comes from it, to heat too much and to spoil very shortly after it was made on account of such heat. Also, when I analyzed the pulp residue, I found most of the valuable elements had not been liberated nor extracted. They were therefore wasted.

Then I tried grating and grinding the vegetables and whizzing the juice out of the pulp in a perforated container revolving at a very high rate of speed, by centrifugal action. This gave me a somewhat better juice, more palatable and easier to make. Nevertheless, there was too much fine pulp in the juice. The pulp residue still contained from 25% to 50% moisture and far too many of the vitamins and mineral elements which were needed in a good and effective juice, were still in that pulp residue. Try as I would, I could not devise any mechanism or means to make a complete extraction by centrifugal action. I finally realized that I was trying to do something which it is physically and mechanically impossible to achieve, namely, the **Complete** extraction of the liquid, and of the elements or particles from any moist material, by centrifugal force.

In the course of these experiments I also tried cutting the vegetables into microscopic particles as fine as dust, hoping that in this way I could get the body to do the extracting. I thoroly mixed these with liquids of different kinds, sometimes water, at other times fruit or vegetable juices. I found however that the fibres of vegetables are too tough for the digestive processes to treat when they are reduced to such a small, fine powder, even when this is wet or moist. Furthermore, I also discovered that frequently in course of time when using too much of such juice, these fine particles would reach the colon and accumulate there until they filled some of the pouches. When this happened, an impaction would follow which would aggravate whatever condition the colon might be in. In such cases I found upon an examination of the feces, that these particles were absolutely unchanged and that they had passed thru the system without the digestive processes being able to work on them on account of their microscopic size. I thereupon discarded this method not only as impractical but also possibly as dangerous to use in trying to make vegetable juices with it.

When, after a great deal of experimenting during many years of research, I finally triturated the vegetables, I found that with the right kind of a grinder I could rip open virtually all of the cells in the fibers and in this way liberate the atoms and molecules they contained. Thanks to Divine guidance and to my innate knack to develop mechanical contrivances, I finally was fortunate enough to develop a triturating grinder which gave me the results I was looking for. Having liberated the elements from the cells of the fibers, my next problem was to collect them in such a way that I could obtain **all** the liquid and **all** the chemical, mineral and vitamin atoms and molecules which it would be mechanically and humanly possible to extract. When I developed a practical hydraulic press in which all these elements could be separated from the pulp, I finally achieved my objective of a complete, effective and efficient juice which would give me consistently the desired results when used according to the combinations and proportions which I found would be most beneficial.

This is the history of the development of the Juicer which, I am happy to say, is now generally accepted as the last word in Juice Extracting Equipment. I have found no other method nor any other machine or device which will give me juices upon which I can definitely depend for the results I seek in helping ailments, sickness and disease, or as a positive means of helping me to **Become Younger.**

The manufacturers of this equipment wanted to perpetuate the recognition of my efforts in these discoveries and wanted to label it with my name, to which I objected. We therefore compromised by their using a neutral name which would include the first few letters of my name, and they called it NORWALK equipment, namely: **NOR**man-**WALK**er. The Manufacturing Company has been given the right to use this name and to manufacture the machines on this principle,

ON CONDITION that the machines would be made to last a lifetime, and so mechanically perfect that their efficiency and operation would require little or no service thruout their life. Another condition was that the machines would be sold at the lowest price possible consistent with the highest grade of material and workmanship, and that under no circumstances would QUALITY be sacrificed to meet any competition which might arise.

Of course all juices of vegetables and fruits are beneficial, in whatever manner they are extracted, within the limits of the efficiency of the equipment used. If the extraction is not virtually complete, then of course the juices are correspondingly deficient and we will have to take larger quantities of them over a much longer period of time. If the juices are properly and completely extracted, however, the benefits and results which we may obtain from them are almost phenomenal. Thousands upon thousands of people the world over have written to tell me they owe their health and often their life to the judicious use of these fresh RAW vegetable juices. Whatever the first cost of the juice equipment may be, it should never be considered as an expense, but rather as an investment. As a matter of fact properly made vegetable juices, to my personal knowledge, have helped to save many thousands of people from unnecessary operations which would have cost from a few hundred to many thousands of dollars besides the perpetual impairment to their health as the aftermath of surgery. They have helped to save many people from an untimely death and I would hesitate even to guess how many thousands from premature old age. On the other side of the ledger, innumerable people who were considered "healthy" have been helped to **Become Younger** by the sacrifice involved in the initial cost of proper juicing equipment.

We frequently use one or two of the so-called "liquifiers" in preparing some of our meals, but never to make vegetable juices. The manner in which we use it is explained in a later chapter on the preparation of salads and desserts.

For the purposes for which we use the "liquifier" we have found it indispensable. I am very sure that your Health Food Store will help you choose the one best suited to your needs.

The use of vegetable juices to help us in ailments which may afflict us has been covered quite completely in the book RAW VEGETABLE JUICES, What's Missing In Your Body? and it would be much better to study that book, than to have me repeat here my experience in the extensive use of these juices during the past 40 or 45 years or more. One or two examples, however, should be given so you may understand the reason for using some juices abundantly, and others sparingly.

Take the condition of peptic ulcers, for example. I used one or two pints daily of fresh raw cabbage juice with perfectly marvelous results, more than 30 years ago, and have never had a recurrence of them. I found, however, that while many others who followed my example derived the same benefits, they complained of a terrific amount of gas. When they changed from cabbage juice to the fresh raw carrot juice, however, they found the results to be even more satisfactory and no excessive gas bothered them. The reason of course is that cabbage contains quite a large proportion of sulphur and other gas forming elements, while the carrot is better balanced in this respect.

Parsley, as you will learn from studying the above Juice book, is a very potent juice and we have found that it should be used very sparingly by itself. In combination with other juices it has been found extremely valuable and beneficial.

Beet juice is another excellent aid. We received this week a letter from a lady in Florida who is in her late 70's. She installed a Norwalk juicer in her home a year or two ago and this is what she says:

"I'm doing lots better with my diseased organs and making good progress, but I had a long way to go, so I'm not yet as well as I'd like to get. I'm still plugging along. I'm now taking lots of beet juice. It makes me dizzy and stirs me up, but I'm now able to keep it on my stomach. For a long time I could not keep it down nor could I relish it. It was positively repulsive to me, but I'm making better progress since I can take it.

"My condition was of such chronic standing that I was a total wreck, in nerves as well as physically. I would not go to an institution that did not treat according to my specifications, for my health's sake, so I've stayed home and plugged along."

You will understand from this letter how important it is to use beet juice, judiciously and intelligently. It is a valuable juice to help us **Become Younger.**

Chapter 22.

IMPORTANT AIDS TO HELP US BECOME YOUNGER.

I do not know whether you were properly impressed with my details regarding the results of starvation of the colon? You will remember that once the walls of the colon have lost their tone thru lack of the nourishment needed to keep the nerves and muscles active, they become flabby. They are then very much like the jacket of a sausage which has only a very little filling or none at all. In this state the colon is likely to droop, to form into loops, or become elongated and seriously interfere with the passage of matter to be evacuated. We call this a prolapsed colon. Any prolapsed organ has the tendency to make the whole body feel as if it were sagging. In the course of a very short time after this condition occurs, there begin, in many cases, to appear lines in the face which cause the mouth, the chin and the corners of the eyes to droop. In any case these prolapses may have a definite depressing effect on the system which has a tendency to make us feel and look old and tired particularly when we have to stand on our feet any length of time.

Some years ago an elderly gentleman in California discovered that, by placing a board in a slanting position, one end on the edge of a stool or a low chair and the other on the floor, and lying on it on his back with his head on the lower end, and his feet on the upper end, he felt much relief from an abdominal pressure of long standing. After using the board for a few minutes at a time, several times a day, he discovered in the course of a few days that he was having better and more natural bowel movements than formerly. In seeking a reason for this improvement he discovered that his prolapsed colon was taking a rest, as he put it, while he lay in that inclined position. This gave it an opportunity to move back into a more natural position, and resulted in a less obstructed passage of waste matter with the consequent improvement in his elimination.

He continued to use his slanting board as a regular daily routine and soon discovered many other benefits he was deriving from it. Among these was a feeling of restful peace which enabled him to get up from the board much refreshed. In course of time, he experienced a sense of rejuvenation, and altho way up in years, he walks, looks and acts like a man well rejuvenated. His slanting board is undoubtedly one of the means which has helped him to **Become Younger.**

We have suggested the use of this board to a great many people, and invariably we have received most satisfactory and gratifying reports as a result of using it.

Besides using this slanting board for relaxation purposes, he uses it also to exercise the whole anatomy. In the inclined position, with the head at the lower end, he raises his legs into the air and moves them in bicycle riding fashion. He also balances himself on his shoulder blades, raising his legs still higher, then moves them way over to one side, then to the other, thus helping to flex his vertebrae and limbering up his whole anatomy.

I consider this slanting board a most excellent means to help prolapsed organs to relax, to help the functions of the colon and as an aid to give invaluable exercise to many parts of the anatomy which we are so apt to neglect in our daily routine of living. By all means, use a slanting board as an aid to **Become Younger.**

A friend of ours who lives in the State of Washington, close to the Canadian border, asked us to send her some information about these boards. Last week we received a letter from her in which she says: "Thanks for slanting board literature. I appreciate it very much. In fact I ordered one right away, as the girls (her daughters) donated a portion of the cost for my birthday gift from them. I am so pleased with it, for now our entire family and friends can share it with me." This friend used the slanting board we have in our home when she was visiting us some months ago.

Many people are obliged to stand on their feet sometimes for hours on end. Often they have such a "gone" feeling in their midriff that they wonder if they can stand another minute. Of course **we** know that this is due to the fatigue resulting from incorrect eating and drinking, and from lack of proper elimination of waste from the system. Nevertheless, many of my students, and many others as well, have derived great benefits from the use of the slanting board to help relieve this strain. By using the board, their prolapsed colon and other organs were given a respite which reacted beneficially on the whole system.

Another aid which has been very helpful to those who would **Become Younger** is a vibratory massage. One particular vibrator which we use in our home has been our constant helper for many years. When properly used, a vibrator can be of immense benefit. Massaging probably was discovered the day primitive man failed to escape his primitive wife's rolling pin when it came in contact with his head. By rubbing the point of contact hard and vigorously he discovered that the pain disappeared and to her amazement he probably brought the rolling pin in contact with **her** head and taught her how to rub the pain away.

Today, when a child hurts itself, mother rushes to rub away the pain, while grandpa rubs his rheumatic knee as hard as he can if the pain becomes too uncomfortable.

In the modern home we find the electric vibrator an indispensable gadget. It is used to massage the scalp, thus stimulating the flow of blood more freely thru the capillaries. In massaging the face and neck it stimulates the activity of the skin.

In cases of sickness or disability a vibratory massage is both helpful and pleasing, but it is well to consult your Doctor before using it, because his knowledge of the anatomy and the effect of massage on the afflicted parts of the body may save trouble and damage to the patient.

Manual massage is hard work, as everyone knows who has given someone a good deep rub up and down the spine or on the muscles of the legs or arms. A good vibrator sets on the back of the hand, vibrating it so that a mere gentle touch of the fingers is reinforced by the energy of the vibrator, adding force, without pressure, and penetration to the vibrating movements of the fingers. This seems to make it possible to help the stimulation of the innermost tissues of the body, as well as the flow of the blood to the skin, without digging the fingers into the flesh. It is thus possible to give to oneself, no less than to others, an effective massage which is relaxing, pleasant and refreshing.

Massage is a procedure which is not employed frequently enough. It is very useful in some acute inflammations, tho in these it must be gentle. It is of great service in the treatment of sprains of joints and fractures of bones.

There are many conditions under which the body may respond quicker to a vibratory massage than if left to take complete rest. When tired, for example, and there is no time for a nap, the vibrator may help

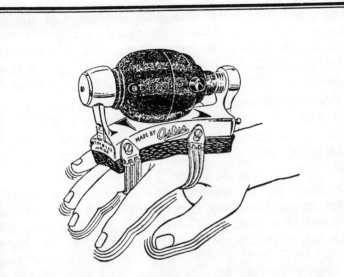

This is the VIBRATOR we use in our home

We chose this one because we found it the most efficient of all those we tested.

Its "suspended motor action" is unique and gives the massaging fingers a rotating-patting movement which is controlled by the pressure of the hand.

With it, the massage ranges from one that is mildly soothing, to one that is deeply penetrating.

It is good for the BODY, for the SCALP, for the FACIAL, for the GUMS and for the FEET. We have found that it helps to make the skin softer and smoother.

It is truly a wonderful help when one wants to BECOME YOUNGER.

to stimulate the system and give us a spurt of energy. After strenuous exercise a vibratory massage is very beneficial, as it helps to increase the circulation to the parts massaged, to dissipate the waste products of fatigue, to soothe the nerves and to relieve tension.

We have therefore found that a good electric vibrator is a very valuable thing to have in the home. There are of course many good ones on the market and no doubt your Health Food Store can supply you with a good one.

I would like to warn against the use of a vibrator in certain specific cases, except under the direction and guidance of a doctor. These are: on wounds and burns, on skin eruptions such as eczema, on blood vessels which are in any way afflicted, on cancerous growths, abscesses and ulcers, acute inflammation of joints, and in pregnancy.

In our experience, a good electric vibrator which leaves the fingers free to do the work, is a very helpful aid to anyone who wants to **Become Younger.**

Chapter 23.

PHILOSOPHY NECESSARY TO BECOME YOUNGER.

Before I give you some menus and recipes to guide you into a change from your old eating habits to the Natural nourishing foods, I want to impress on you the need of developing a very definite philosophy if you would **Become Younger.**

The first principle of this philosophy is RIGHT THINKING. I have said a great deal herein about positive and negative thinking and talking. I want to go into a little more detail regarding this, so that your life may blossom out into a more beautiful experience that you ever dreamed could be yours.

Gossip is the lowest form of pastime unless it is constructive. Never criticize or think evil of others. Think only of the GOOD in them.

We cannot think evil of others unless there is evil, or the spark of evil, within ourselves. To think and to speak evil of others simply lays bare some evil in our own character, whether we realize it or not.

Never pursue an argument when you see the other party will not be convinced or converted. It is better to lose an argument and retain a friend, than to win an argument and to lose a friend.

When we are listening to a person speaking, whether in a lecture or in the home or elsewhere, and some constructive advice is being given, don't let your mind wander to all the people you know who could profit from that advice. Apply it to yourself, first. We are so prone to want to correct and improve others,

177

overlooking the fact that probably we need the correction and the improvement more than anyone we know.

There are critical times in the life of every man and woman. Never talk about your troubles, adversities, hardships or afflictions except on the rarest occasions when your experience may be helpful to your listener. People are not interested in YOUR troubles. They are too much engrossed in themselves.

A downcast demeanor, with a frown, dejected eyes and a droopy mouth, invites old age to visit us and repels the sunshine of life. Lift up the corners of your eyes and of your mouth, and smile, smile from the heart, smile as if you mean it, and before you realize it you will be smiling from the very joy of living. Nothing lifts one up, and others, too, as a constant perpetual smile. A smile can make us see the humor of the most aggravating situations, and humor is an attribute of youthfulness. A smile can lift the burden of woe and self pity, and it does not cost anything to smile.

Happiness, peace and security are sought by everybody. These cannot be found outside of ourselves. Until we have found and developed them within us, within our heart and mind, we will continue to seek them in vain. Once we have discovered how easy and simple it is to find these in our own consciousness, we get an entirely new perspective of life. We can then readily appreciate how worth while it really is to **Become Younger.**

When we embark on this program which requires usually a complete change of our eating, drinking and living habits, we are nearly always confronted with the opposition of our family and friends. This is something we must learn to take in our stride. To face and combat such opposition we must have the courage of our convictions based on the knowledge which we can acquire thru study and practice of the principles involved in this program. We will always find more people ready to tear down and condemn, than to help and encourage. Once we have made a start and begin to feel and express the surge of new life, energy and youthfulness, our assurance that we are on the right road to **Become Younger** should give us the means to combat any negative opposition we may be faced with from those who know nothing whatever about the discovery we have experienced.

To **Become Younger** means to have attained a state of sublime self-reliance and self-sufficiency which no one can take away from us. A state in which nothing whatever outside of ourselves can affect us. Only then can we be Master of ourself and Master over every situation.

Chapter 24.

FASTING.

This is a very appropriate subject to cover before we learn how to put together a meal.

Fasting is a very important part of any program related to the human body. It is very beneficial, PROVIDED that it is done intelligently and not prolonged for a longer period than 6 or 7 days AT THE UTMOST, at any one time.

The effect of fasting is two-fold. It gives the digestive system and a great many of the body functions a more or less complete rest, and at the same time it enables the body to burn up and eliminate waste.

During a period of fasting the body uses its reserve supply of elements to keep the system functioning. It is exceedingly important to know this and to remember it when we embark on a fast.

During a fast we eat no food whatever. We drink large quantities of water or **fruit** juices somewhat diluted with water. This dilution is necessary because otherwise the burning up of debris in the system becomes too severe or concentrated. Fruits are the cleansers of the body, and, particularly during a fast, they must be used with discretion, altho we may take as much fruit as we want, with benefit, at other times.

The amount of such liquid taken during a fast has usually been not less than 2 quarts, but preferably one gallon or a little more thruout each day of the fast.

Such a fast usually has the effect of stirring up a great deal of the waste matter which has been allowed to accumulate in the system. Some of it passes out of the system in the regular course of evacuation and elimination. Much of it, however, is simply stirred up and lodged in some convenient niche or recess, usually in the sacculations or folds of the colon. If allowed to remain there overnite, we are apt to absorb some of the toxins or poisons which this debris may produce. This would have the tendency to defeat some of the benefits we expect to derive from the fast and may also cause some discomfort and excessive amounts of gas. We therefore take a high enema each night of the fast, just before retiring for the night, using the strained juice of two lemons in the water, as given in detail in a previous chapter

At the end of the time chosen for the fasting period, we "break" the fast with two or three light meals consisting of fresh vegetables or fruits and plenty of vegetable juices, for the first and second days, then we resume our normal course of nourishment.

If we have in mind taking a **prolonged** fast, we take it in series of fasts and "breaks". We will fast for about 6 days, then "break" it for 3 or 4 days as indicated in the preceding paragraph. We will then start the fast again for a similar period, with a similar "break" at the end of the 6th day, and so on, as long as we feel we need to continue.

It is an exceedingly dangerous and harmful procedure to fast, without interruption, over a longer period than 6 or 7 days at a time. If we do, the body gets no opportunity to replenish its reserve supply of elements and goes on burning up first the debris, then cells and tissues, without new material to repair or restore these.

There is no question that a prolonged fast without such "breaks" every 6th day makes one feel superlatively exalted, but this exaltation is derived at the expense of the burning up of the body, a condition which does not manifest adversely sometimes for several years.

There was a Doctor with whom I was well acquainted, who placed his patients on a citrus (usually orange) juice fast for 3 and 4 months at a stretch. I pointed out to him the danger of this practice, but he was so well satisfied with the quick results his patients obtained that he would not agree with my arguments. In the course of my lecture tours thruout the country, however, I had occasion to meet a great many of his patients, many of them bedridden, who were seeking some help for their "mysterious" malady. Without exception, they were apparently perfectly healthy, but they seemed to have not one atom of energy in their system. A review of their past history and experience brought to light the fact that they had taken these prolonged fasts and considered themselves cured of what ailed them, but in the course of time, ranging from two to five years, their vitality, strength and energy began to ebb very fast and unexpectedly.

It required many months, in some instances years, to overcome, by means of fresh vegetable juices and a nourishing raw food diet, the damage done by such fasting.

I have right here before me now the X-ray picture of the colon of a lady who was afflicted with cancer, according to the medical reports some 5 or 6 years ago. Lumps began forming unexpectedly in her breasts, on her arms and in other parts of her body. She read about some successful treatments by means of a grape juice fast, and decided to try it. After about 6 weeks of fasting, the lumps began to disappear and she began to feel better than she ever felt before. She continued the fast, unbroken, for another few weeks, then went back to her former three meals a day. There was no apparent indication that any of her ailment remained and she continued happily on her way and in her household duties, with more zest than she had experienced in many years.

About two years ago the full impact of her prolonged fast struck, and struck hard. She could not get out of bed, she became nervous to the point of hysteria, and even daylight upset her until her room had to be kept in semi or total darkness. Her mind was gradually becoming affected and her family and relatives became very much alarmed.

She was finally placed on a rigid Natural raw food diet, which included several pints of raw vegetable juices daily. Twice every week she was given the best colonic irrigations she could get. In less than 6 months' time her whole condition improved very close to the healthy normal. When I saw her recently she looked 5 years younger than she did when I first saw her 6 months previously. Her skin, which was sallow and lack-luster, is now colorful, radiant and sparkling with health.

Not everybody is able to get the meticulous care and family cooperation which this lady was fortunate enough to have. It enabled her to pull out of a dangerous situation in a much shorter time that I would have thought possible. This merely proves that where there is a will, there is a way.

Let us bear in mind, therefore, that while brief periods of fasting may be beneficial and help us to **Become Younger,** prolonged fasting is definitely harmful, if not dangerous.

Chapter 25.

"NATURAL FOOD" MEALS.

My interpretation of NATURAL FOODS is that food which is nourishing by virtue of the presence of organic life in it. In this category I place all raw vegetables and fruits and their fresh, raw, unprocessed juices, and nuts.

Among the vegetables I would include some of the legumes when they are fresh and young.

Dried legumes lack essential organic water and I have found are too acid forming in the system to be of practical benefit. We therefore do not use them. In this class we include dried peas, beans, soy beans, peanuts, and their many products and by-products.

Whenever possible, we use food that has been grown in or on organically cultivated ground without the use of industrial chemical fertilizers. This is something that is vitally important to understand. Deficiency of vitamins and elements in food is the result of the destruction of the soil by these chemical fertilizers. A few people in the Government are beginning to wake up to this realization.

Organic gardening means the rebuilding of the soil by means of the biological transformation of vegetable and animal wastes into top-soil thru the life processes of soil organisms such as earthworms, bacteria, etc. Only in this manner, the manner adopted by Nature since vegetation began on the face of the earth, can we produce a fertile and productive ground on which to grow food with an abundance of vitamins and minerals.

Vegetables and fruits grown on such soil need no poison dusting nor spraying. Under such circumstances insects and pests do not destroy crops, as the birds in the natural course of events feed on them. Birds are the best and most efficient insect destroyers, and they are utterly harmless. One family of chickadees, nuthatches or titmice can wipe out more than 80 **pounds** of insects during a single summer, while a few pairs of titmice can eat up all the tent—and other caterpillars and flying insects on one single acre of apple orchard. A pair of swallows and their family can feed on about 7,000 flies in a single day. A chickadee can destroy as many as 5,500 canker-worm moth eggs in one day.

What happens when vegetables and fruit trees are sprayed? Birds eat the poisoned insects and die. Insecticides are thus responsible for a great deal of the increase in pests and insects and the consequent damage to food. Insecticides kill only a few pests, compared to those existing all around, and by their destruction of birds also, they defeat their own purpose, as the insects and caterpillars are then able to propagate and multiply outside of the poisoned area without interference from the birds! In Morristown, N. J., a whole flock of wild birds was found dying of convulsions at the same time, and a pitiful number fell dead out of the trees when these were sprayed.

Honey is our most valuable carbohydrate food and sweetening. Scores and hundreds of beehives have failed to yield a supply of honey because the bees died of insecticide poisoning.

Without industrial chemical fertilizers, but using organic gardening principles instead, and fostering the growth of earthworms in the soil, we can get not only much larger crops but also far superior products, and after all it is the quality of the food we eat that will help us to **Become Younger.**

The finest quality Irish potatoes have been harvested at the rate of 1,000 to 1,200 bushels to the acre while carrots have been grown at the rate of 100 to 105 tons to the acre on organically prepared soils. The quality of these vegetables made the finest vegetable grown on the chemically fertilized ground look like culls and scrub.

An organization was formed not so long ago, known as the SOIL & HEALTH FOUNDATION, with headquarters at 46 S. W. Street, Allentown, Pennsylvania. If organizations such as this could spring up all over the country, we would soon be able to get the quantity and the QUALITY of food that the whole of the United States of America needs, to **Become Younger.**

While we are not always in a position to choose the quantity and the quality of the vegetables and fruits we need, we can to a great extent overcome this handicap by drinking plenty of fresh raw vegetable juices of as much variety as possible.

As for our daily meals, supposing I give you an outline of what my own meals consist.

For Breakfast: 1 or 2 ripe bananas. These have no green whatever showing, and preferably with as much brown in the skin as possible. Ripe bananas are an excellent food. Cut out any spoiled parts, after removing the skin. Slice thinly, or mash with a fork in a soup plate or other deep dish.

Carrot pulp. We have a Triturator, so I triturate about 2 or 3 teaspoons of pulp, **without** squeezing out the juice. Failing a triturator, use an Acme or similar grater (described in the book DIET & SALAD SUGGESTIONS) and grate the desired amount of carrot pulp. Spread this over the banana.

186

Raisins. I prefer the seedless. Soak some overnite in cold or tepid water. Spread 2 or 3 teaspoonfuls of these over the pulp.

Figs. The black Mission figs are my favorite. They are dried, so, soak some as you did the raisins. Cut the stem off and slice 4, 5 or 6 over the entire dish.

Nuts. We use a Norwalk Nut Grinder with which I can grind unsalted almonds almost as fine as flour. I spread about 4, 5 or 6 tablespoonfuls of these finely ground almonds over the whole dish, and that is my breakfast. If you do not have such a nut grinder, your Health Food Store can probably advise you what to do about it, or may be able to supply you with them.

Should you so desire, you could use some cream, preferably raw cream, to moisten the food. If so, put it on before spreading the nuts.

A glass of carrot juice or of potassium, or even one of carrot and spinach, gives me the best drink I could want.

You will be amazed to find how thoroly satisfying this breakfast can be.

There are many ways in which it can be changed and varied. Using the banana as the base, a sliced or coarsely shredded apple or pear, with raisins and figs as indicated above, with or without the rest of the ingredients, makes a delicious and delightful breakfast.

Personally, I find this the most satisfying breakfast of all. In fact I doubt if I have changed my menu more than half a dozen times, just once or twice each time, during the past several years. After some practice I believe that you, too, will find in these suggestions the answer to the kind of breakfast that stays with you, without the discomfort of gas.

Lunch depends on circumstances. If I happen to be away from home at lunch time, I take with me some fruit, such as apple or pear, or other fruit in season. Some celery and a small avocado, if one is available. Otherwise I may take—occasionally—a small amount of swiss cheese. This food, together with a pint or two of fresh vegetable juices, gives me all the nourishment I need till dinnertime.

If I am at home, however, I eat a small salad consisting of a variety of vegetables. For example:

In a soup dish I may place 2 or 3 teaspoonfuls of carrot pulp. Over this I spread some finely chopped up celery, green onion, cabbage or lettuce, and a little green pepper, mixed together. Over this I spread some dressing, any one of those I shall list in a few minutes.

Next is about 2 teaspoonfuls of finely shredded beets. I add about a tablespoonful of raw green peas over all, and place a small piece of raw cauliflower in the middle. Of course you can season it to your taste with some vegetable salt, which by the way you can also obtain from your Health Food Store. Apply the seasoning sparingly on each layer.

With a glass of vegetable juice, this makes a very satisfying lunch for me, which does not leave me tired and hungry before dinnertime.

It only takes a short time to make such a salad. If you will remember that all vegetables will mix in a compatible manner, and you have the choice of chopping them fine or coarse, grating them fine or coarse or shredding them, as the case may be, with a little practice you can make a variety of salads with exactly the same vegetables, just prepared differently. In fact you will be amazed at the simplicity with which either a simple or an elaborate meal can be prepared.

Any one of the vast number of menus and recipes which I have put in my book DIET & SALAD SUGGESTIONS, is well balanced and subject to a profusion of changes which will give you quite a variety in appearance and flavor. It simply means preparing each vegetable in the way best suited to your taste or to the time you have available to prepare it, chopped, sliced or grated.

One of the secrets of making a good salad is to mix 2 or 3 vegetables per layer, and use 2 or 3 layers for a salad. This will give you an infinite variety to choose from. Do not use too much of any one vegetable.

The dinner meals are just as simple to prepare and can be made as simple or as elaborate as one desires.

One of my favorite implements for salad making is our Liquifier. It helps to break up the fibers of the vegetables and makes them somewhat more palatable, PROVIDED the switch is operated EXACTLY as I say, and that the vegetables are not allowed to be broken too fine by the switch being left on for more than ONE SECOND at a time. Work it thusly:

Chop up some celery with a sharp knife on your chopping board, say about 2 tablespoonfuls, and put them in the Liquifier bowl. Add enough liquid just to cover the knives completely. This liquid should preferably be carrot juice or the juice of any green vegetable. If none is available, some fruit juice (unsweetened) will do, otherwise some plain water can be used. Chop up about 2 tablespoonfuls of lettuce, the same way you did the celery, and put it on top of the celery. Cut up a tomato into several pieces and add to these. Place the top cover on, and turn the switch on but immediately turn it off again. **When the knives have stopped spinning** push the mixture down with a spoon then turn on the switch and immediately turn it off once again, and—be sure the knives have stopped spinning—push the mixture down once more. Repeat this as often as needed to break up the vegetables as fine as you want them, but not "liquified". Do this over and over, a dozen times or more if necessary.

Next, strain the liquid from it and you have your first mixture ready. You can either use this as the first layer of your salad, or you can put about 2, 3 or 4 teaspoonfuls of carrot pulp in a soup dish and spread the mixture over it, adding a little vegetable salt for your seasoning.

Pour the strained liquid from the above mixture back into the Liquifier to make your next layer. Take 3, 4 or 5 green onions and cut them up into fairly small pieces using also about 2 or 3 inches of the green part. If you have no green onions, any other onions will do instead. Put this in the Liquifier. Grate about a tablespoonful of cucumber on the coarse grater, peeling and all, and add this to the onion. Cut up finely about a tablespoonful of green pepper and add this to it. Chop as finely as possible about a tablespoonful of cabbage and add it to the other ingredients. Add some vegetable salt to flavor, and repeat the process of turning on the Liquifier for one second at a time, turning the switch on, then immediately turning it off, as often as necessary to have the cabbage as fine as you want it.

Strain the liquid off this mixture and it is ready to add as the next layer. Here you can inject a variety of changes. For example, you can peel an apple and grate it coarsely on the coarse grater, and spread about 1 or 2 tablespoonfuls over the mixture on the dish before adding the cabbage mixture, then add this mixture evenly over the apple. Instead of apple you could use a pear or any other fruit or berries that appeal to you. It is entirely a matter of taste, and what appeals to me you may not like, and vice versa. So do some experimenting and even if you should strike some mixtures that do not appeal to your taste, they may not do you any harm but on the contrary may be quite nourishing, altho of course you can change them next time.

So, we place the grated apple on the dish and on it we spread about 2, 3 or 4 tablespoonfuls of the cabbage mixture over it. Next, we get out the fine grater and grate about 1 or 2 tablespoonfuls of raw beet, which we spread over the cabbage mix. We sprinkle a little vegetable salt over this, then squeeze about a teaspoonful or less of lemon juice over the beet. We garnish this with a ring of green pepper about ¼ inch or less in thickness, in the center of which we place a sprig of cauliflower and around the latter we place a few slices of red radishes.

Of course if you do not happen to have a Liquifier this does not prevent your making exactly the same salad with the same mixtures. It just means cutting, chopping or grating the various vegetables to the consistency that practice and your tastes will dictate.

Throughout the preparation of this "layer type" of salad you can use whatever vegetables and fruits you have available using the same general principle in your method of preparing it. As a matter of fact you will rarely need to sit down, chew the end of your pencil and say to yourself: "Let me see, what shall I use today?" Just get your vegetables out of your refrigerator and take them as they come or as they appeal to you, and with a little practice, before you know it you may be able to make a real masterpiece of a salad.

You have no idea how much this way of eating simplifies housekeeping. You know what a mess it is to stack up a lot of greasy, dirty dishes, to have to wash them and almost if not thoroly sterilize them, then have to clean off the grease from the sink! Our method of eating does away with nearly all that mess. In fact:

191

Say—Great Scott and Little Fishes—
'Tain't no job to wash the dishes.
Tell you how:—I shouldn't ought'er—
I just rinse them in hot water!

Dressings for salads can be made as tasty as they are nourishing. Use the same ingenuity in concocting your mixtures, bearing in mind NEVER to use vinegar nor pepper. Vinegar, you know, is really acetic acid and may have the tendency to burn the membranes of the digestive tract. Ulcers may develop quite readily from the use of vinegar. Pepper and similar strong condiments may have a like effect on the system. Do not be misled by the habits of taste. When you see people who are apparently in the pink of condition, who have been eating their meals with plenty of vinegar and pepper interspersed here and there, just watch for the appearance of ulcers and also for many indications that Old Man Time is sharpening his scythe, or may be just the sickle that cuts off youthfulness at the roots, leaving the rest to wither.

Olive oil is available nearly everywhere. Mixed with honey and lemon juice, it makes a very nourishing dressing. We never use sugar. You may add a little vegetable salt if you wish.

Try this for a superlative dressing:

1/3 cup olive oil; 1/3 cup lemon juice; add 3 or 4 medium size tomatoes, ¼ teaspoonful of vegetable salt and ½ to 1 teaspoonful of honey.

Mix these in the Liquifier for about 2 minutes. Add about ½ clove of garlic if you are going to use it right away, otherwise put it in a mason jar and put 2 whole cloves of garlic in to flavor, without breaking them up.

A good avocado dressing is made by peeling it, removing the seed and cutting up the avocado into small pieces in a bowl. Add a little hot water, about ½ teaspoon per avocado, and mash with a fork. Chop a few green onions into it, add about ½ teaspoon of honey and a little vegetable salt and beat it up either with the fork or with an egg beater. If you want to, you may add one or two teaspoons of sour cream, or sweet cream with the addition of a little more lemon, for each avocado used.

Never forget that any starch or sugar taken during a meal in which lemon or any other acid fruit is used, will create acidity in the system.

I have not given you here a variety of menus, because you can find a mass of them to suit every occasion, in my book DIET & SALAD SUGGESTIONS. It will be much simpler for you to use that book, than to have to study them out of this larger book.

Desserts can be as delicious as they can be mystifying when made in a Liquifier. For example: Put about a cupful of carrot juice in it. Add a banana cut up in large slices. Two heaping tablespoonfuls of ground unsalted almonds. 2 or 3 heaping taespoonfuls of soaked raisins. 3 or 4 soaked figs. 2, 3 or 4 tablespoonfuls of cream. Whip this up in the Liquifier for about 2 minutes or more. Serve this in a dessert dish, with some whipped cream if desired.

NOTE:
Read the chapter on VINEGAR in my book RAW VEGETABLE JUICES, What's Missing In Your Body?, the Revised, Enlarged 1970 Edition. It recommends the use of APPLE CIDER Vinegar only and tells you WHY!

Chapter 26.

Let's BECOME YOUNGER Together.

In conclusion I want to warn you that to **Become Younger** is a slow process, requiring patience and perseverance. You can become aged overnite, but you cannot **Become Younger** until you have undone the harm to your body which has resulted from a whole lifetime of wrong eating, wrong living and wrong thinking.

Wrong eating means eating and drinking anything whatever that fails to furnish the cells and tissues of the body with LIFE. As we cannot have life and death at one and the same time, and excessive heat— that is to say, heat in excess of 98° to 105° F. temperature— destroys the life in our food, it is obvious that, while cooked and processed foods enable us to sustain life, they do so at the expense of the complete regeneration of our body. They cannot furnish LIFE to the body. That must come from the raw vegetables and fruits and their fresh raw juices.

To overcome a great deal of the necessary time or period of rejuvenation, we have found that fresh raw vegetable juices, properly made from good quality vegetables, help to speed up the process. The greater the speed with which we want to rebuild the body, however, the greater may be our reactions. Therefore we must have an understanding of this process and of these reactions, and above all, we must never become discouraged. Nature works in mysterious ways. When we give Nature the implements to work with, and submit ourselves without reservation to Her ministrations, She will not let us down. She may find more things to correct in our system than we have any idea of, but if we will trust Her to correct everything in turn, she will do a marvelous job for us, and She will help us **Become Younger.**

Let us bear in mind, then, that to indulge our appetites and desires without regard to their final outcome may set us back every time. Do we want the satisfaction of the moment, at the cost of grief, sorrow and regrets later on? That is the question that every one of us must answer for himself, every time.

Wrong living means living or existing thru life without an intelligent purpose or aim. We cannot live for ourself alone, altho the I is the most important element in our existence. Unless we take care of ourselves first, foremost and last, we cannot be of any good or value to ourselves nor to anyone else. Therefore our first consideration MUST begin with ourself. The care and attention we give to our physical mental and spiritual body will reflect our value to the rest of the world. If we neglect to care and develop our own trinity, our physical, mental and spiritual system, we will soon become useless to ourself and to the rest of the world. We will be heading for senility and the discard. We must learn to live, and at the same time give all we can of our physical, mental and spiritual gains for the benefit of others. Only by giving do we grow. When we study, intelligently, we grow in knowledge, and when we spread that knowledge, judiciously, we are amazed to find that we gain more and greater knowledge.

Knowledge is like the seed of plants. Keep it tucked away, and the seed is eventually worthless. Plant it, cultivate it and nourish it and the whole neighborhood will gaze at and enjoy the splendor of your flowers. These in turn will bring you more seeds, because you made good use of the first. Tithing is the most outstanding example of this principle. Keep to yourself all you make, and you will just plug along thru life, may be or may be not able to make ends meet. Give 10% or more of what you make, as a tithe to something worth while, and almost as if by magic your abundance will increase. Therefore remember that with knowledge as with everything else, we must GIVE, in order to receive.

Wrong thinking means holding, keeping or developing thoughts that are not constructive, thoughts that are negative. No truer saying was ever given to mankind than: **As a man thinketh in his heart, so is he.** And don't think this applies to **man** alone. It means **woman** just as much.

If we could only live a life in which we see no evil, we do no evil and we think no evil, most of our troubles would vanish.

As we part, for the moment, let me leave these thoughts with you:

Do not judge the contents of this book from your own knowledge of what to eat and what to drink. I have merely given you in these pages what I know from my own personal knowledge, experience and observation. Its contents have been known, consciously or subconsciously, since the beginning of time. My researches lead me to know that anything to the contrary is the result of man's folly and frailty. The knowledge of Nature's laws, only a fraction of which it is possible to give in these few pages, is indestructible.

Do not lay this book away for the silverfish and mice to eat its paper. That is the only thing that is perishable about this book. Its printed word is indestructible, and you may want to refresh your memory now and again, so leave it where you and your family and your friends can see it and maybe get a mite of benefit from some word or sentence or page herein that I have placed in your keeping.

Remember that when you talk, you repeat what you know. When you read and when you listen, you very often learn something.

An empty box makes a lot of noise when there is only one pebble in it, but when it is full, it is silent and weighty. It is the same with the human head.

I shall never forget what I heard when I was a boy 18 or 19 years old. It was one of the milestones in my career:

"The more you think you know, the more you'd better listen".

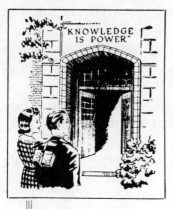

If anything in this book has given you pleasure, benefit or happiness, write it down and let us know about it. It matters not whether this is your book or if it is loaned to you. This is the only way we can know that our work has been profitable to the reader.

We will appreciate it, even though it is only a post card with one or two words and your name and address on it.

Dr. N. W. Walker's Books
may help you rejuvenate body and spirit

With so much confusion these days about what to eat, and why, and how to cope with the spiritual and emotional problems of our times, these timely books by Dr. WALKER are needed in every home. He is a living, dynamic example of his teachings.

BECOME YOUNGER (for all ages)
You are Never too Old!
RAW VEGETABLE JUICES
What's Missing in Your Body?
VIBRANT HEALTH — The Possible Dream
WATER CAN UNDERMINE YOUR HEALTH
YOUR FOUNTAIN OF HEALTH
Your Pocket Guide to Juices

2-COLOR WALL CHARTS — 17" x 22"
(Suitable for Framing)

Colon Therapy	Endocrine Glands	Foot Relaxation
What you MUST know about YOUR Colon.	What DO You know about your Glands?	Used extensively in ZONE THERAPY.

ALL AVAILABLE AT MOST HEALTH FOOD STORES

MAIL YOUR ORDER TO:

NORWALK PRESS, Publishers
2218 East Magnolia
Phoenix, Arizona 85034

199

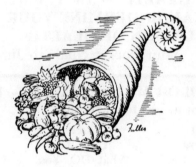

INDEX